FORMULATION

as a Basis for Planning Psychotherapy Treatment

FORMULATION

as a Basis for Planning Psychotherapy Treatment

Mardi J. Horowitz, M.D.
Professor of Psychiatry
Director, Center on Stress and Personality
Langley Porter Psychiatric Institute
University of California, San Francisco, California

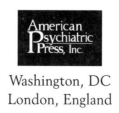

Washington, DC
London, England

Copyright © 1997 American Psychiatric Press, Inc.
ALL RIGHTS RESERVED
Manufactured in the United States of America on acid-free paper
First Edition   00   99   98   97   4   3   2   1

American Psychiatric Press, Inc.
1400 K Street, N.W., Washington, DC   20005

Library of Congress Cataloging-in-Publication Data
Horowitz, Mardi Jon, 1934–
     Formulation as a basis for planning psychotherapy treatment / by
Mardi J. Horowitz. — 1st ed.
       p.   cm.
     Includes bibliographical references and index.
     ISBN 0-88048-749-6 (alk. paper)
     1. Psychiatry—Case formulation.   2. Psychiatry—Differential
therapeutics.   I. Title.
     [DNLM: 1. Psychotherapy—methods.   2. Patient Care Planning.   WM
420 H816f 1997]
RC473.C37H67   1997
616.89—dc20
DNLM/DLC
for Library of Congress   96-35388
                                                                      CIP

British Library Cataloguing in Publication Data
A CIP record is available from the British Library.

Dedicated with grateful appreciation to all the people who, in the midst of distress, gave consent to participate in clinical research, in the hope that others, in the future, might benefit.

CONTENTS

INTRODUCTION

As clinicians, we hope to help our patients with accurate diagnoses and effective treatment plans. In this effort, we must first identify a patient's most salient problems and then devise a plan for addressing these problems. Such plans often involve psychotherapy with goals ranging from the reduction of symptoms to the prevention of relapse. In addition, we often want to help our patients recognize and remove impediments to more effective functioning, because failures in functioning will exacerbate anxiety, depression, and rage.

Diagnosis alone does not complete this process. Treatment plans based only on descriptive classifications, such as those of DSM-IV (American Psychiatric Association 1994), do not necessarily target changes in root causes. Formulation fills a gap that would otherwise exist between diagnosis and treatment. With an adequate system for formulation, we can plan individualized treatments.

All trainees are taught some system of case formulation, yet many clinicians are dissatisfied with what they learned (Goldsmith and Mandel 1969). Some clinicians have been taught formulation systems from different schools of psychotherapy and are then expected either to use them eclectically or to arrive at a personal integration. I have come to believe that a systematic approach should be based on an integrative effort. The system presented here combines concepts derived from psychodynamic, interpersonal, cognitive-behavioral, and family system approaches.

The system I present focuses specifically on planning effective psychotherapy with the concomitant use of medications and social interventions. This formulative approach is embedded in a biopsychosocial model and focuses on an individual's personal psychological meanings, emotions, and coping efforts in that model (Engle 1980).

To use psychotherapy to facilitate processes of personal change, a patient usually must reflect on personal meanings by gaining knowledge, altering irrational or dysfunctional beliefs, and experimenting with trying out new modes of thinking, planning, and acting. These changes in beliefs and behaviors may need to be integrated with previously segregated aspects of personal meanings, such as various roles of identity and previously dissociated or contradictory intentions, goals, and values. By learning and practicing new behaviors in therapy, and in the social world of work, friendships, and love, the patient learns new ways to resolve long-standing dilemmas. The patient also may learn new ways to compensate for biological limitations, social stigmatizations, and psychological sequelae of past traumas and deprivations as well as inevitable future frustrations. Formulation can point out what needs to be done to meet such goals. My focus on the psychology of personal meaning includes an effort to understand the current biological and social contexts in which change processes may take place.

After an overview of psychological change processes in Chapter 1, each of the five steps of the formulation process are covered in the subsequent chapters. In Chapter 2, I explain how to begin a case formulation by the careful selection and description of a patient's symptoms and problems. In Chapter 3, I organize this information by describing how selected phenomena can be grouped into states of mind, a key strategy in this system for integrative case formulation. In Chapter 4, I explain how to interpret all of this information to infer important themes that can provide a treatment focus and to identify defensive controls that may interfere with treatment. In Chapter 5, I provide ways with which to infer deep beliefs about the self in terms of views of relationships with others. In Chapter 6, I cover plans for interventions during psychotherapy.

Start With the Present, Shape the Future

The action of psychotherapy is aimed at improving present and future functioning. Although it may, at some point, be important to explore the past to find out how and why patterns were formed, we ground our inferences on present observations. For example, a person may be demoralized by the lack of good working relationships with peers and impeded by argumentativeness. How and why argumentativeness developed in childhood family interactions is important to formulate, but not until the present pattern is selected and clarified as the target of our efforts at explanation.

Clarification of the present is not easy. Defensive compromises between wishes and fears often obscure the situation. In fact, defensively avoidant styles may have become character traits. By repetition, the trait is both automatic and often invisible to the person who has the trait. Formulation involves seeing through such opacity to deep-seated dilemmas within the inner world of memory and desire.

Such obstacles may impede the discovery of how deep-seated dilemmas cause the repeated maladaptive behavior patterns and symptoms of conscious distress reported by a patient. Complex layers of action and emotion combine with contradictory attitudes to cloud understanding. Wish-fear dilemmas and conflicts between expressive and defensive aims also lead to confusing signs. As I explain the formulation process, I address these issues and how they can be worked through.

In writing this book, I had my own dilemma. The book is meant for a beginner in the fascinating career of a clinician. Usually, such beginners learn most from their supervisors, who are well versed in one or more schools of formulation. My integrative focus involves the use of different terms than those used by some supervisors. Establishing the historical evolution of this integrative system would require a longer text, but trainees deserve a short book. Because the logic of my approach has been published elsewhere, I selected the latter choice.

Clinicians face a similar dilemma when formulating a case during early evaluation and treatment. The formulation must balance the simple and complex. If a formulation is too simple, it can overlook important knots that need to be unraveled. If a formulation is too complex, it only muddies efforts to think clearly about how to help. Our goal is a "just right" level of complexity. I believe a *states-of-mind* approach helps us to achieve this balance. It allows for multiple presentations of a patient rather than insisting on too-static descriptions of observations, yet it also simplifies many observable features into meaningful clusters of co-occurrence.

A states approach allows us to discuss motivation with a patient in terms of how desired states are related to dreaded states and how certain states are intended to function as ways to avoid confrontation with relevant emotional issues. Thus, we can deal with a "configuration" of wish, fear, and defense as a simple and direct approach to current concerns.

We can examine configurations surrounding any aspect of self, whether it is a lifelong dilemma, an unresolved memory, or current stress-precipitating psychiatric symptoms. I use diagrams to present and clarify such configurations of complex cases. These figures allow us to grasp the interacting concepts all at once, not just in prose sequences that must address concepts in a linear fashion. Throughout the book, the figures are easy to follow because I use the same spatial layout.

I argue that the systematic approach taught in this book helps condense a great deal of information into tentative explanatory models. This task, however, is neither quick nor easy. Resist anyone who demands that a finished formulation need not be subsequently modified; that is unrealistic. Only a provisional, tentative formulation can be made so early. Revisions and elaborations should occur as more information is obtained and as psychotherapy progresses. Early formulations are partial, incomplete, and sometimes wrong. Formulation is like making sense of a puzzle; just stay with it, and the pieces of information will eventually fall into a pattern you did not notice before.

ACKNOWLEDGMENTS

Many ideas about emotional conflicts involving wishes, fears, and defenses stem from S. Freud (1900, 1903, 1912a, 1912b, 1913, 1914, 1923). His formulation of what was happening beyond a patient's immediate conscious awareness included configurations of wish, anticipated and feared consequences of expressing wishes, and defenses to ward off those consequences. Many additions and revisions have occurred since Freud. These are synthesized into an approach called configurational analysis.

I use the term *configurational analysis* to label a multiview examination of the interplay of wish, fear, and defense and various structures of knowledge and belief. I derived this term from Henry Murray (1938) and Erik Erikson (1954). I used *configurational analysis* as a label for an individualized approach to the formulation of problems, defensive stances, and alternative concepts of identity and relationships in different states of mind of an individual (Horowitz 1978).

To use an integrative language that allows discourse across disciplines, I made a major effort to select words in discussion with other psychiatrists, psychologists, anthropologists, neuroscientists, and psycholinguists. Convergence of terminology evolved from a series of interdisciplinary workshops encouraged and supported by the John D. and Catherine T. MacArthur Foundation. The evolution of this language is reported in a series of books (Horowitz 1988a, 1991; Singer 1990). I thank all these colleagues.

The emphasis on observing and selecting key phenomena for subsequent explanation rests on the shoulders of Karl Jaspers (1968) and DSM teams led by Robert Spitzer (DSM-III [American Psychiatric Association 1980]) and Allen Frances (DSM-IV [American Psychiatric Association 1994]). My addition has been a states-of-mind approach (Horowitz 1979/1987, 1988b) that regards observable discords and inconsistencies in experience and behavior as meaningful patterns rather than noise. My work on states, and the varied self-concepts of any individual, followed the concepts of Jung (1939), Janet (1965), Federn (1952), Berne (1961, 1964, 1972), Gaarter (1971), Piaget (1930), Bartlett (1932), Allport (1955), and Ashby (1952, 1960).

As reviewed theoretically elsewhere (Horowitz 1988a; Horowitz et al. 1994b), state cycles are important to observe and may occur, in part, because of changes in defensive control processes. The related theory of *control processes* (Chapter 4) has been based both on psychoanalytic investigators such as Anna Freud (1936) and George Vaillant (1993) and on cognitive scientists such as Rumelhart and McClelland (1986), Benjamin and Friedrich (1991), and Stinson and Palmer (1991). Attention and action control theory is central to this modern view of defensive control processes (Horowitz and Becker 1972; Kuhl and Beckmann 1985). What I present in Chapter 4 is consistent with what is currently known about both psychological and biological processing of perceptions, ideas, and emotions (Dixon 1981; Ekman and Davidson 1994; Horowitz 1991; Kosslyn and Koenig 1992; Lazarus 1991; Posner 1989; Singer 1990; Uleman and Bargh 1989; Wegner and Pennebaker 1992).

The relational approach to self and other beliefs and schemas in Chapter 5 stems from S. Freud's (1905, 1912a) work on transference and later additions by psychodynamic investigators (Luborsky 1984; J. Perry 1991; Strupp and Binder 1984), object-relations theorists (Fairbairn 1954; Greenacre 1952; Kernberg 1975, 1976; Klein 1948; Winnicott 1953), self psychological theorists (Basch 1973; Gedo and Goldberg 1973; Kohut 1977; Lichtenberg 1975), control-mastery theorists (Weiss and Sampson 1986; Weiss 1995), and the schemas and pathogenic belief work of cognitive theorists (A. T. Beck 1976, 1987; J. S. Beck 1995; Kelly 1955). The present integrative approach is part of a modern convergence of psychodynamic and cognitive-behavioral theories (Beitman et al. 1989; Horowitz 1988a, 1988b, 1991; Kurtzman, in press; Stein, in press).

My contribution, whatever its worth may be, would have been impossible without 10 years of excellent support for risk-taking empirical, clinical, and theoretical work. For this, I am deeply grateful to all involved in the Program on Conscious and Unconscious Mental Processes (PCUMP) of the John D. and Catherine T. MacArthur Foundation. I am especially indebted to Charles Stinson, M.D., Constance Milbrath, Ph.D., Bram Fridhandler, Ph.D., Mary Ewert, Ph.D., Alan Skolnikoff, M.D., Norman Mages, M.D., Tracy Eells, Ph.D., George Bonanno, Ph.D., Steve Reidbord, M.D., Are Holen, M.D., Nigel Field, Ph.D., Henry Markman, M.D., Sandra Tunis, Ph.D., Dana Redington, Ph.D., Jerome Singer, Ph.D., Lester Luborsky, Ph.D., Christopher Perry, M.D., Howard Sherrin, Ph.D., Zindel Segal, Ph.D., Susan Andersen, Ph.D., Peter Salovey, Ph.D., Michael Bond, M.D., Steven Cooper, Ph.D., Jess Ghannam, Ph.D., Tom Merluzzi, Ph.D., Daniel Hart, Ph.D., Gordon Bower, Ph.D., Stephen Palmer, Ph.D., Wilma Bucci, Ph.D., Helena Kraemer, Ph.D., Robert Emde, M.D., Matthew Erdelyi, Ph.D., Paul Crits-Christoph, Ph.D., Peter Knapp, M.D., John Conger, Ph.D., Charles Marmar, M.D., Dianna Hartley, Ph.D., Bryna Siegel, Ph.D., Daniel Weiss, Ph.D., and many others involved in PCUMP.

I began working on this manuscript as a Rockefeller Foundation Scholar at the Bellagio Study Center and finished during a fellowship year at the Center for Advanced Study in the Behavioral Sciences (itself partly supported by the MacArthur Foundation). Kathleen Much and Julia Salzmann provided essential editorial input. Nancy Kaltreider, M.D., Leonard Zegans, M.D., Robert Nemiroff, M.D., Marc Jacobs, M.D., and Adriana Feder, M.D., all affiliated with the University of California at San Francisco residency training program, provided highly useful pragmatic advice by reading various stages of the manuscript. Residents in my seminars fueled the effort. Other invaluable input was contributed by faculty and trainees during my visiting professorships to Harvard University, Stanford University, George Washington University, University of Washington, and the University of California at Los Angeles.

I am deeply grateful to the patients who participated in our research and, thereby, enabled the work to happen. All case examples use fictitious names and have other altered features. Julia Salzman and Gerald Richards were superb in editing the manuscript and shaping its figures.

Chapter 1

FORMULATION FOR PSYCHOTHERAPY

We begin formulation with a clear description of problems. Later, we develop explanations of why they have been hard to solve. We use these explanations to establish goals of psychotherapy and strategies to reach those goals. The goals involve changes in the patient that can endure after treatment ends.

The question of what *can* change is an important one. In this chapter, we examine some preliminary answers and give a quick overview of an integrative approach. We also begin to examine ways in which formulation can be used to determine treatment.

What Can Change?

The patient can change dysfunctional beliefs and behavioral habits, especially irrational beliefs about how the self relates socially to others and inhibitions in life activities and self-development that exist because of excessive fear or inappropriate despair. The patient can also reappraise past memories and fantasies and reconsider future goals. Areas of confusion can be clarified. Plans can be made and carried out with support. Contradictions may be integrated, and conflicts resolved. Incomplete mourning can be completed. Self-concepts based on realistic and competent skills can be developed.

Modifications of this sort often increase life satisfaction and reduce anxiety and depression. Many patients, however, confront "damned-if-you-do and damned-if-you-don't" dilemmas that typi-

1

cally stem from social conflicts and biological disturbances. These dilemmas then live on in the mind as contradictory systems of belief and emotion. Negative moods and diffusely focused attention and information processing can impair functioning. Change can be facilitated by evaluating mood and neural substrates for information processing. Social supports and aids can help the patient add rational or functionally adaptive beliefs to counteract irrational or dysfunctional ones. Psychological interventions can facilitate new integrations of previously discrepant ways of experiencing personal identity and social relationships.

Patients can learn how to accept unalterable conditions when necessary and establish achievable personal goals for the future. Hope and morale can be restored. Mental capacities may be increased. Patients can learn to use their minds as tools to help them function more purposively. Treatment aims at mental growth that can compensate for unalterable liabilities as well as the alteration of changeable pathologies.

Course of Therapy

Our first goal in therapy is the stabilization of the psychology of the patient and any surrounding biological and social circumstances to reduce risks to self and others. A closely related first aim involves reducing symptoms and distressing but prolonged moods. An ethically grounded, expert therapist can help a patient develop trust and incentive for further change. We encourage realistic aims for treatment outcome. In developing a good relationship, we demonstrate an understanding of problems and a path for arriving at a focus for the treatment. Motivation to change and realistic hopes of success in treatment help the patient to reduce states of fear and despair.

Then, in the middle phases of therapy, the patient may be enabled to make new choices. Gradually, instead of automatically repeating symptom-formation cycles and habitual avoidances, the patient learns new activities, confronts personal dilemmas and unresolved topics, attempts new relationship experiences, and experiments with new self-attitudes. A greater continuity of personal meanings evolves. Finally, a patient accepts termination of the treatment and the supportive relationship with the therapist.

Obstacles to Change

Human beings find unsolvable problems unpleasant to consider. If past personal efforts and prior treatment have failed to help matters improve, why repeat the distress by focusing on impossible dilemmas? Patients reduce displeasure by avoiding topics that cause anguish. Avoidance also reduces the risk of acting impulsively and then having to face bad consequences. Change in psychotherapy involves recognizing and modifying such avoidances.

Different therapy techniques use different strategies to direct attention toward usually avoided topics. Formulation helps define these ideas and feelings. The patient may have so habitually avoided confronting enduring problems, however, that averting attention from them is automatic. If you direct attention to warded-off topics, your patient may, in the safe relationship with you, be able to think the usually unthinkable and speak the usually unspeakable.

A patient may carry into the therapeutic relationship various relationship beliefs and motives. A yearning for love, an expectation of scorn, or a grudge may color a patient's view of any relationship, including the one with you. Irrational expectations may arise and lead to various frustrations and fearful withdrawals. Wanting unselfish caring, a patient may also expect love followed by abandonment. Patients may test you and their relationship with you to see just how safe or unsafe a relationship can be in this new situation.

The beliefs the patient may test with an individual therapist or within a therapy group will usually be based on real or fantasized experiences within past relationships. The experienced transactions within these past relationships become schematized in the mind. The patient asks, in effect, is this new context like or unlike these schemas? Might this new, present circumstance be an opportunity to act on my intentions to satisfy my innermost intense desires? Might this new present circumstance lead to enactments of my worst fears? Is the apparent safety of the therapeutic alliance transient or stable, true or false, resilient or brittle? Is my therapist ethical and professional or a sham, a quack, a manipulative exploiter? Such fears can be obstacles to working for personal change.

The patient may learn from these tests whether transferred inner beliefs about self and others are justified in the current context. If your relationship in therapy seems dangerous, then the patient will continue to avoid direct expressions of personal dilemmas, deep worries, and usually warded-off wishes and fears. If the context seems safer than past situations, then avoidance may be reduced and tentative expressions may begin. Step by step, a sense of safety evolves, and obstacles are bypassed.

Selecting a Focus

Why should patients contemplate topics that have negative emotions? Most people will be willing to face them only if they see hope of a better outcome than before. If there is a chance of getting "safe help," they will contemplate a difficult topic. Contradictory attitudes and antithetical beliefs may then be considered.

It is important for beginning therapists to realize that a patient may express *both* trust in you *and* an expectation of betrayal from you. This is an example of contradictory beliefs about the same person. Allowing contemplation of such contradictory beliefs can clarify for the patient his or her recurrent patterns in maladaptive relationships.

Within the focus on personal meaning systems and plans for how to act in life, a patient may change by 1) developing more rational views and action patterns; 2) modifying styles of habitual avoidance of certain areas of contemplation and behavior; and 3) learning to use new rational views and behavioral styles that can either counteract or contain irrational views and prior, impulsive patterns of behavior. Small changes accrue and lead to larger, slower, and more difficult changes. As a patient tests for safety, and finds it (Sandler 1960), he or she is likely progressively to confront more and more emotionally complex topics. Increasingly, conscious control processes will be used to modify habitually nonconscious defensive operations as well as prior patterns of poor coping with impulses.

In this manner, the focus on complaints and problems begins to include the causes of these symptoms. The patient examines beliefs and goals and learns how to handle deficits and integrate discrepancies and contradictory views about self. New ways to evaluate the self as having these concerns are developed. New ways to work, gain intimacy, or improve caretaking functions are evolved. The new patterns of action may feel awkward at first, but adaptive behaviors have more rewards than maladaptive ones. A patient can be motivated to repeat them. Each repetition gets less awkward, and, eventually, the patient acquires poise and deftness where once he or she had problems.

Some patients first try out new ways of behaving with the therapist. Some model new behaviors based on the ways the therapist deals with the patient's problems. Others engage directly in new activities simply by deciding to use suggestions offered by the therapist. Others combine all of these routes to a change in functional capacity in the domain of focal attention.

Cycles of Therapist Activity

The therapist facilitates the patient's efforts to change by directing attention in useful ways. Therapists are sometimes relatively passive (carefully listening) and at other times relatively active (speaking). Formulation helps therapists to oscillate between listening and speaking in an expert way rather than a random or improvisational one. There are many occasions for intuitive intervention, but formulation allows for systematic intervention. A cycle of expert passivity and expert activity is shown in Figure 1–1.

The activity of the therapist in the *expert passivity loop* of Figure 1–1 begins with *free-floating attention* to observing the patient. Attend not only to the words spoken, but also to the verbal and nonverbal communications and your own emotional and imaginative responses. Free-floating attention allows you to mix objective and subjective responses to the patient and leads at times to the useful intuitive responses mentioned earlier. It is valuable to balance this free-floating deployment of attention with *focused attention*. Focused attention involves mini-formulations. It allows you to choose rationally how and when to intervene. It prevents you from blurting out sudden intuitive insights that will not, at this point, help the patient. Careful listening consists of a useful oscillation between free-floating and focused attention.

Most of the time, this loop refers to the time you spend in session with the patient. But focused attention to phenomena and their causes

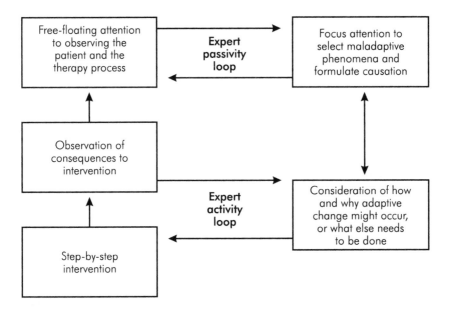

Figure 1–1.   One possible cycle of therapist activity during the middle phase of psychotherapy.

is appropriate outside of sessions, when you can concentrate without distractions. When the case is confusing or difficult, and when routes to progress seem blocked, formulation outside of sessions is imperative. Time for reflection should be included in any institutional arrangement.

As you develop formulations during periods of focused attention, aided by useful intuitive "ah!" experiences, you can plan treatment interventions. The operations of implementing these plans are the *expert activity loop* of Figure 1–1. You act and then observe how your patient responds to the intervention. If the results are as expected and a change occurs, then you can return to listening. If the results indicate something other than you expected, you may reconsider and revise the intervention. Revising an intervention may be very important when a patient misunderstands your messages or intentions.

Cycles of Patient Activity

By the middle phase of psychotherapy, a focus and sense of safety has been established. Patients learn to report more and more frankly

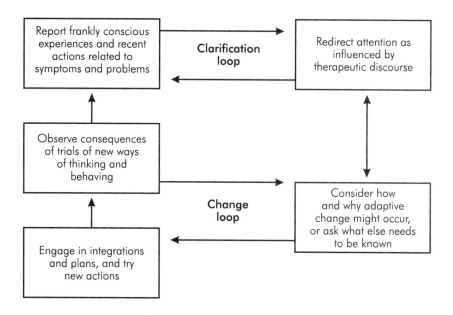

Figure 1–2. One possible cycle of patient activity during the middle phase of psychotherapy.

their conscious experiences and recent actions related to the treatment focus. They set aside some fantasies of how therapy might work in favor of realistic goals for learning, making, and practicing changes that reduce problems and symptoms as well as strengthen capacities. In this middle phase, there are cycles of patient activity that can be called loops of clarification and change.

A patient's frank reports of conscious experiences and recent actions begin the loop of clarification. As a consequence of how you listen and act, the patient will redirect attention. This cycle leads to additional frank reports. The process continues until a maladaptive behavior or dysfunctional belief is sufficiently clarified to warrant efforts to change it. At that time, the patient shifts into a loop of change (see Figure 1–2).

Change processes may include conceptualizing more adaptive beliefs or behavioral patterns, or considering what else must be known. Once possible activities are clarified, patients engage in these activities. They may form integrative beliefs or act on plans for more adaptive actions.

Next, patients observe the consequences of their new activities. This may lead to a reconsideration of what to change and a repetition through the loop of change. The consequences of revised activities are observed. Once the consequences of new behaviors and thoughts have been observed and found satisfactory (for the time being), patients return to the clarification loop.

Overview of Five Steps of Formulation

The steps of formulation are summarized in Table 1–1 and explained in each ensuing chapter. These steps begin at the surface and continue to deeper inferences about what causes the selected phenomena. Your emerging formulations will guide your treatment plans, and your constant modifications of these formulations will guide your expert activity during therapy. The utility of formulation is both macro- and microanalytic, and the convergence between the two has been demonstrated empirically (Horowitz et al. 1993b, 1994b).

First, select *phenomena* for explanation. These may include clusters of symptoms, unresolved life choices, or maladaptive interpersonal actions. Next, consider the *states* in which the symptoms frequently occur. Good questions may spring to mind: Do some situations evoke problem-filled states? Are there desired states that are seldom or never achieved? When and why do state transitions occur? State cycles may be examined. Then describe *defensive impediments* to therapy. As defensive obstacles are reduced, the final two steps are more readily achieved. In the fourth step, *identity and relationships*, you clarify maladaptive patterns of interpersonal behavior and problems with loss of self-esteem. Once important beliefs about self and others are listed, you can ask more questions: Are there discrepancies between belief and consensual reality? Are there contradictions in beliefs and real opportunities? Do dilemmas between wishes and fears paralyze action? Finally, in the fifth step, you relate the four preceding levels and plan how change may occur or how to find out what you still need to know.

Other useful questions include biopsychosocial linkages. How did the person learn his or her states, roles, transactional expectations, and style of defense? From whom? Are there available but unused

Table 1–1.   Steps of formulation at the psychological level of the current situation

Phenomena

Select and describe symptoms. Determine what problems need to be explained.

States of mind

Describe states in which the selected phenomena do and do not occur as well as recurrent maladaptive cycles of states.

Topics of concern and defensive control processes

Describe themes of concern during problematic states. Describe how expressions of ideas and emotions are obscured. Infer how avoidant states may function to ward off dreaded, undermodulated states.

Identity and relationships

Describe the organizing roles, beliefs, and scripts of expression and action that occur in each state. Describe wish-fear dilemmas in relation to desired and dreaded role relationship models. Infer how defensive control processes and compromise role relationship models may ward off such dangers. Identify dysfunctional attitudes and how these are involved in maladaptive state cycles.

Therapy technique planning

Consider the interactions of phenomena, states, controls, and role relationship modes. Plan how to stabilize working states by support, how to counteract defensive avoidances by direction of attention, and how to alter dysfunctional attitudes by interpretation, trials of new behavior, and repetitions; integrate psychological plan with biological and social plans, when indicated.

Note.   Each step can also include social and biological levels as well as past developmental contributors to the current situation.

strategies for improved coping? At the biological level, are there disturbances among or within neurotransmitter and neuronal networks that make state stabilization and optimal thinking difficult to achieve? Are there social factors that increase vulnerability to lapses in control?

The phenomena selected at the first level continue to be revised as states, defensive control processes, and role relationship models are formulated. If a habitual defensive control style of avoiding serious expressions, for instance, by joking about emotional topics, is formulated at step 3, this might lead back to noting a trait of difficulty in expressing emotions to others back at step 1. Bantering may then be

Table 1–2.	Domains of formulation

Psychological domain
   Present aspects
   Developmental aspects
Social domain
   Present aspects
   Developmental aspects
Biological domain
   Present aspects
   Developmental aspects
Co-determination
   Present aspects of intercausation
   Developmental antecedents of intercausation

Note. For possible inclusion as an aspect of each step of Table 1–1.

recognized as a state at step 2; being a joker may become a role of self entered at step 4. Observations latent in your memory may become active and help to clarify concepts as a result of systematic formulation efforts (S. Perry et al. 1987; Strupp and Binder 1984).

Organization of Formulations

You can use subheadings at each step of formulation. These subheadings can link current perspectives to developmental antecedents and can link psychological, biological, and social factors. This kind of organization is shown in Table 1–2. In this book, I focus on psychological formulations with "open door" examples showing how to describe and integrate social and biological features. This system allows you to condense information and revise inferences as you obtain more information.

Process Notes

Formulations often stem from your review of process notes that record your impressions following the completion of a session with a patient. A systematic format for process notes may be helpful; an example is provided in Table 1–3.

Now, a case formulation is illustrated. The purpose of this example is to give a rough, preliminary, and therefore incomplete sketch of the whole approach before we engage in the more detailed, chapter-by-chapter, step-by-step exposition.

☐ Case Example: Mr. Silver

Mr. Silver was a 31-year-old unmarried man when he sought treatment for anxiety symptoms. He had felt generally tense for many years, but in the last 6 months he had periods in which his tense muscles, sweaty palms, sense of dread, and preoccupation with worries interfered significantly with his work. He was diagnosed 3 months earlier as having a generalized anxiety disorder and treated with antianxiety medication. The drugs reduced his symptom levels, but he and his primary care physician felt he should discontinue the medications because of the danger of their long-term use. That decision led to referral for psychotherapy.

Mr. Silver had worked for several years at a low management level in a large corporation. He had been promoted about 6 months earlier. His increasing responsibilities involved more frequent and important interactions with the people whom he supervised and the people who supervised him. In addition, he had to cooperate more with his peers. The interactions were desirable, but made him feel even more tense than usual. His anxiety symptoms had increased since the promotion.

Mr. Silver desired friendships and intimacy, but seldom had either. Whenever he sought to develop a friendship, he ended up feeling rejected and unworthy. Having learned that he did not do well socially, he tended to stay away from people. This withdrawal did not quite reach the criterion for a diagnosis of social phobia. He could make himself be in a group, but tended to feel very alert to possible signs of scorn, rejection, or exploitation by others.

He often felt very dissatisfied and restless. He wanted to have more pride in his products and to be able to share excitement more with peers at work. He wanted more intimate friendships and sexual companionship, even to get married, but he seldom could feel joy or even relaxation with others.

Table 1–3.	A format for psychotherapy process notes that help formulation

Therapist: _____

Patient: _____

Date: _____

Session: _____

A. **Summary of interview**

B. **Summary by categories**

   1. *Events since the last interview* (include main topics of concern and changes in phenomena):

   2. *States of mind* (include observed and reported states of the patient, states of the therapist, and patient-psychotherapist as "we"):

   3. *Topics of concern and defensive control processes* (describe conflictual topics and obstacles to clarity and therapeutic work):

   4. *Identity and relationship beliefs and interpersonal behavioral patterns* (include current, past, and imagined future aspects of pathogenic beliefs):

   5. *Formulations, plans, and major interventions* (acts of the therapist and their effects on the patient):

At work, he hoped to develop cooperative partnerships with peers. He felt uneasy and suspicious, however, that they would be too competitive and dislodge his chance of advancement in the company. If they tried to get closer in cooperation, he felt edgy and would back off from them, feeling more anxious about whether he was doing the right thing or the wrong thing. He would go back and forth, approaching them and avoiding them.

A recent relationship with a woman gave him hope. They had sexual relations and dated for 3 months. When he asked her to move in with him, she ended the relationship firmly but kindly, saying he was "not right for her." He felt she viewed herself as superior to him and did not see him as worthy of a domestic partnership or marriage. He had dated a few times since then, but felt the women involved were not the sort of person he wanted to stay with.

As a result of limited closeness of relationships in both his work and his love life, he sometimes felt lonely and sad. He would listen to music, which he loved, to ease his distress. He would drink alcohol in moderation.

During evaluation interviews, he was initially engaging, clear, and appropriately seeking help. After the opening phases of each session, he then seemed to slump down and draw back and say he was unsure about being there. Then he would alert himself and try to come out of his shell. He checked on how he was being received by the clinician. He expressed feelings, and yet he also made efforts to suppress them. The feelings, flickering over his face, seemed to be a mixture of self-disgust, sadness, and fear.

Phenomena

As the first step of formulation process, we can list Mr. Silver's phenomena as worries about the intentions of others and frequent anxious tension that resulted in tense muscles and sweaty palms. These complaints were more distressing when Mr. Silver was with people. By avoiding people, he could usually feel numb rather than anxious. Avoiding people kept him from satisfactions he desired: joy, excitement, togetherness, and pride in being with an effective group. If and when he tried to get closer to people, these interactions often led to feeling degraded, sad, lonely, and shameful of being unwanted.

Mr. Silver's phenomena included his presenting complaints of anxiety. He avoided people to reduce this problem, and avoidance itself was a problem. His goal of sharing with others was not satisfied, and he had a problem of chronic rejection. The aim is to understand more about these problems and how to modify them.

States

Mr. Silver's anxiety symptoms occurred in a tense state of mind. This tense state contrasted with a dull state, achieved and stabilized when he could work by himself in his cubicle. He did desire a state he called happiness. He differentiated happiness from a state that he sometimes experienced with great distress, one of feeling shamed by rejection, lonely at his lack of relationships, and sad that this condition seemed unchangeable. This state felt degraded. A configuration of these states is found in Figure 1–3.

The configuration of states shown in Figure 1–3 follows a format that is repeated in future examples. The format begins with presenting complaints, as in the upper-left corner of Figure 1–3. Presenting symptomatic states, such as that of tension in Mr. Silver, may sometimes function as initial concerns. These initial concerns may not include a patient's need to alter deeper concerns, such as Mr. Silver's dread of entering an intense, degraded, and shame-filled state shown in the lower-left corner of Figure 1–3. With efforts at restoration, the person may reach better states, with fewer problems or symptoms. These are called quasi-adaptive, reading over to the upper-right quadrant of

Problematic compromise	Quasi-adaptive compromise
• Tense apprehension	• Dull loneliness
• Degraded shame	• Joyful intimacy
Dreaded	**Desired**

Figure 1–3.   Configuration of states for Mr. Silver.

Figure 1–3. I call this quadrant "adaptive" because it contains fewer symptoms and problems, and "quasi" because the experiences are not as satisfying as the patient may desire. A search for something more is found by reading down from the upper-right quadrant to what lies beneath: a desired state. The reason why the goal of joyous intimacy was defensively averted or compromised into tense apprehension or dull loneliness is understood by reading further to the left to find a related threat: his anticipation of degraded shame if he was rejected.

Thus, the relatively raw form of a wish-fear dilemma occupies the deep part of this format or configuration of states. Compromises derived from attempted and partial solutions occupy the surface of the figure. More pleasant or tolerable emotions are generally depicted to the right, more unpleasant or intolerable feelings to the left. Compromises in the upper-left include symptoms like anxiety; less symptomatic but still avoidant solutions to dilemmas occupy the upper-right quadrant. The whole is a configuration of a wish-fear dilemma and possible defensive compromises.

Mr. Silver had a cycle of states. He would seek closeness at work or in a social situation. Because of his previous patterns, he would anticipate rejection and feeling degraded. He would then get tense as he forced himself to approach others. While engaging them with as much charm as he could muster, he was also anxiously alert to their possible lack of interest or exploitation. His hypervigilance to rejection would win out, and he would wall himself off from others. Again, he would feel alone in his dull state of mind. This cycle is illustrated in Figure 1–4.

Themes and Defensive Control Processes

Mr. Silver was in danger of degraded states. He was afraid rejection would lead to loss of self-esteem. When these issues came up, he spoke disparagingly of others in a way that dislocated his inferior attributes onto them. He could, by this reversal of roles, reject others from a superior posture. He could wall them off without a sense of a lost opportunity. He could switch to focusing on how to develop his own interests by concentrating on work or listening carefully to music while alone. The switch in roles of relationship or from relating to others to a self-preoccupation is modeled in Figure 1–5.

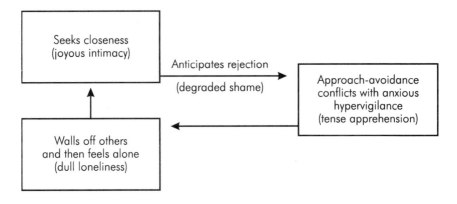

Figure 1–4.   Cycle of states for Mr. Silver.

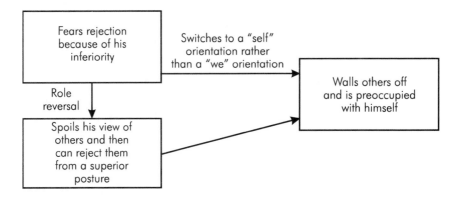

Figure 1–5.   Defensive control processes for Mr. Silver.

Identity and Relationships

Mr. Silver's repeated stories allowed me to infer a role relationship model for each of his states. By switching between these beliefs about self and others, he could accomplish his defensive reversal of roles. That shift in his defensive control processes then led to his state cycle.

His wish to become happy was linked to a hope to find a really great woman or man friend, a person who would see him as competent and join in mutually enjoyed activities. This goal-related role relationship model is shown in Figure 1–6. This model of the desired happy state is also shown in the "desired" lower-right quadrant of Figure 1–7. Unfortunately, when Mr. Silver sought closeness with a companion, he feared that the other would be too superior and so reject him. He would recoil in sadness and shame, entering a degraded state of mind, as shown in the "dreaded" lower-left quadrant of Figure 1–7.

To ward off the danger of the dreaded, degraded state, he defensively reversed the role for self. He occupied the aggressor role of superior companion, seeing the other as unworthy of his attention. He was then suspicious and rejecting. Yet he had a sense of his own defensiveness and felt tense and anxious about losing an opportunity for a good relationship. That problem-filled compromise role relationship model organized his experiences and interpersonal actions during his tense states of mind and is shown in the upper-left of Figure 1–7.

In a less symptomatic state of mind, he avoided others. He viewed himself as sufficient unto himself, and this seemed to include grandiose beliefs in his stature and skills. Others were uninteresting, and he walled off any approaches they might want to make toward him. While telling himself he was superior, he still felt dull and numb, but that was better than tension and better than intense sadness and shame. He still desired closeness, and that desire might trigger another

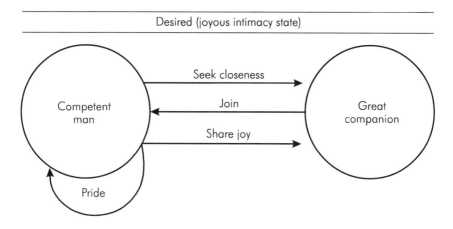

Figure 1–6.   Role relationship model for Mr. Silver.

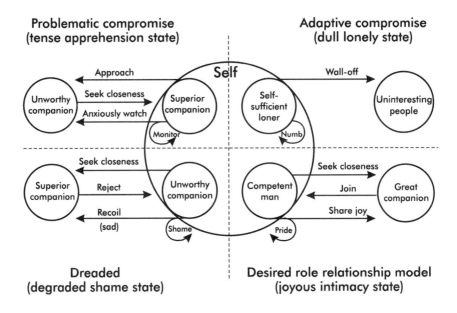

Figure 1–7.   Role relationship model configuration for Mr. Silver.

cycle of seeking others, feeling about to be rejected, rejecting others, and withdrawing. This quadrant of a quasi-adaptive compromise completes the configuration shown in Figure 1–7. It resembles in format the configuration of states and phenomena given earlier in Figure 1–3.

Mr. Silver had self-concepts of both grandiosity and inferiority. Unfortunately, he did not seem to recognize and integrate these alternatives. He did not have an overarching sense of identity. He experienced only the identity of the state he was in at the time. This limitation resulted in a dysfunctional imperative, a pathogenic belief that "I must be superior or I will be inferior and rejected; if I am not superior, I am scared of being left alone."

Implications for Psychotherapy for Mr. Silver

The fifth step of formulation leads to a plan for treating Mr. Silver. The description of his phenomena leads to a plan to supply clear labels for sharing during the exploration of what situations, internal or external, may trigger his problematic experiences. That would permit better recognition of what causes symptom formation. Identifying these triggers will help him stabilize less anxious states. Knowing his potential states will also help the therapist be alert for the negative effects of treatment, such as entry into dangerous (potentially suicidal) states of shame, depression, and hopelessness if confrontation with difficult topics proceeds too rapidly.

After state stabilization, the reasons for Mr. Silver's maladaptive state cycles could be addressed. With insight, he could consciously work to modify his tendency to wall himself off from others. Instead of his usual approach to gain relief from tension, he could experiment with other ways of coping that did not result in so much loneliness. Mr. Silver could be encouraged in realistic ways to engage more in feared situations. His role reversals and withdrawals could be noted in his reports of such engagements with others. Then he could learn how these defenses functioned to blunt his negative emotions.

His wish-fear dilemma could be addressed at the level of his major dysfunctional beliefs and contradictory attitudes. He could be helped by discussing various ways to understand and handle rejections. He could be engaged in discussion of ways to seek closeness that might be more socially effective. The irrational components and sources of his unworthy self-concepts could be challenged. More rational views of self and more skill development could be encouraged.

New behaviors could gradually evolve for cooperative working and gradual courting. Existing beliefs about self and relationships could be better integrated, leading to a more realistic and continuous sense of identity. In the course of such work, Mr. Silver's therapist would be alert for the possibility that recognizing problems and dilemmas could increase his sense of depression. The therapist should be alert to any signs of depression and work with the patient to reinforce signs of hope and zest for life. These aspects of technique are summarized in Table 1–4.

Before Formulation

Obtaining a psychiatric history should precede formulation. This will result in a diagnosis and should follow standard procedures. This re-

---

Table 1–4.   From formulation to technique (Mr. Silver)

Phenomena

Arrive at labels for problematic experiences.

Encourage attention to specific events and contexts that either evoke or dispel symptoms.

States

Stabilize well-modulated "working" states for dealing with difficult topics.

Identify state cycles (hypervigilance to rejection leading to walling off, longing for attention, seeking attention, then being too worried about closeness).

Defensive controls

Identify avoidances and their functions.

Encourage engagement in feared situations.

Clarify how, when, and why role reversals occur.

Identity and relationships

Challenge belief that he has to be superior or else he is inferior.

Model how to handle rejections and how to seek closeness.

Challenge irrationally unworthy self-concepts.

Encourage realistic and positive self-attributions and "closer" behaviors.

---

port should include the reason for evaluation, the course of the present illness, and a biopsychosocial history. Social, occupational, and familial events and a review of moods and other sources of discomfort should be included as well as the results of a mental status examination. Physical examination, diagnostic tests, and psychiatric signs in the interview process should also be recorded before working on cohering elements into an overall formulation.

Approaches to Formulation

The sketch of Mr. Silver quickly illustrates an approach to formulation. Each step is discussed in subsequent chapters with more information on how and why to do it. The preliminary view of how psychotherapy works, given in this chapter, is deepened in the last chapter. Here, on the basis of the sketch so far, we can consider briefly how this approach to formulation compares with others.

In *Psychiatric Case Formulations,* Sperry et al. (1992) reviewed prior approaches. They agreed that a DSM-IV (American Psychiatric Association 1994) (or ICD-10 [World Health Organization 1992]) Axis I diagnosis is, in and of itself, a poor basis for a treatment plan. They presented four major orientations to formulation: the biological, psychodynamic, behavioral, and biopsychosocial integration points of view. They used a historical approach in the chapter on psychodynamic formulation, covering id psychology, ego psychology, object relationship psychology, and self psychology.

The approach you will learn in this book is simpler than that presented by Sperry et al. (1992), although it seeks answers to the same questions. What are symptoms and why do they occur? When do they first occur and what perpetuates them? The reason I say this approach is simpler is that it does not require that trainees learn several psychodynamic languages mentioned above—ego psychology, object relationships psychology, self psychology—in a historical perspective, and then also acquire other languages from behavioral and biological points of view. Instead, an integration of psychodynamic, cognitive-behavioral, and interpersonal perspectives is used for the psychological component of case formulation. The trainee is not expected to do the integration: it is provided in the system. The result is a scaffold on which the trainee can later construct a wider array of knowledge.

Although the approach is integrative, it includes a psychodynamic attention to configurations of desired goals, dreaded consequences or external pressures, and defensive avoidances of anticipated threats. This attention to defensive layering adds to the common approach (across cognitive, interpersonal, and psychodynamic schools of therapy) to the identification of personal, pathogenic beliefs.

In the examination of dysfunctional beliefs, the approach is like that of A. T. Beck (1976) and Persons (1993) in cognitive-behavioral theory. In its attention to self and other responses to initial motives and expressions of intention, this approach is like the core-conflictual-relationship-themes interpersonal approach of Luborsky (1984). In its attention to cycles of varied identity experiences and typologies of behavior, this approach is like the cyclic maladaptive pattern formulation of Strupp and Binder (1984), the multiple ego states approach of Berne (1961) in transactional analysis, the multiple possible selves views in object relations (Kernberg 1975), and the self psychological (Kohut 1977) approaches, as summarized by McWilliams (1994).

In its system for inferring wish-fear dilemmas, and defensive postures in relation to these dilemmas, this approach is like the plan formulation method of control mastery theory (Silberschatz et al. 1991; Weiss 1995; Weiss and Sampson 1986) and the wish-fear-defense formats advocated by S. Perry et al. (1987), C. Perry et al. (1989), and Caston (1993). This system, presented as simply and briefly as I can, was based on the study of these various other systems and grew from these strong resources into a format that combined the best elements of each. In every step discussed in the next five chapters, some aspects of the system to be presented have been checked in quantitative and qualitative empirical studies of recorded evaluation and psychotherapy sessions.

Summary

The goal of this book is to teach a hypothetical trainee to go beyond diagnosis to the kind of formulation that helps facilitate adaptive change in psychotherapy, combined with social and biological interventions. Our view will be mainly toward briefer psychotherapies and cases where extended information may not be available at the time treatment must be started.

In the next chapters, five steps are covered: 1) describing the phenomena chosen for further explanation; 2) examining the states of mind in which these phenomena do and do not occur; 3) observing for conflictual themes and defensive control processes that may obscure relevant information; 4) inferring core pathogenic beliefs as varied and possibly contradictory identity, relationship, and value experiences in different states; and 5) planning treatment in terms of answers to the question, "what can this patient change now?"

The approach is integrative. It emphasizes psychological components because it is a method directed at planning how to intervene in psychotherapy. It includes places to integrate biological and social inferences and strategies. It emphasizes a current approach to causation: what causes and what keeps symptoms going? Yet it includes places to integrate developmental perspectives on how current causal factors originated in the past.

Chapter 2

PHENOMENA

When I was in medical school, we learned how to take a history, do a physical examination, and write up thorough case reports. One of my teachers once made fun of a fellow student who took the detailed outline we were to follow in doing our writeups literally. When the student described the patient's ear canal, he wrote, "No beans present," because the outline had listed beans as one of the things one might find lodged in an ear canal. My heart went out to the student ridiculed so cruelly, but the vivid lesson remained in my memory. Clinicians agree that the art of describing phenomena consists of selection as well as keen observation (Lazare 1973, 1989; S. Perry et al. 1987; Turkat and Wolpe 1988).

Although a patient's chief complaints are always paramount, a list of phenomena goes beyond them. A good clinician needs to select and describe whatever else requires explanation and treatment. Inability to function well is as important as symptoms of distress.

We do best if we regard a list of phenomena as open ended. We can modify it during a course of treatment. I usually begin with *symptoms, signs* I observe, and *problems in living*. Then, I may add topics of concern, topics that seem conflictual but unresolved. These topics may stem from traumatic events or situational crises that threaten the patient.

Symptoms

Many of us tend to emphasize symptoms that form the official basis for diagnoses in the existing nomenclature, DSM-IV (American Psychiatric Association 1994). We tend to be less attentive to symptoms that are not listed in the menus of complaints that serve as criteria for diagnosis. I find it helpful to remember that these menus represent the compromise positions of committees of experts who argued about formal properties of each of the diagnoses. Individual patients may exhibit many more clinically salient symptoms.

Signs

Include relevant signs that you observe in mental status examinations and during psychotherapy. Disturbances in cognition or memory are examples. Signs include observations that a patient's communication contains striking discords. For instance, we may see a momentary facial expression of profound sadness while a patient reports feeling fine, or a fist clenched in anger while the patient is speaking of having a good relationship with a spouse or co-worker. Discords may indicate specific unresolved topics.

Problems in Living

Problems in living go beyond symptoms. Some patients seldom have especially depressed or anxious moods but are distinctly impaired at work, in intimate social relationships, or in caring for children. It may be important to list a patient's unrealized desires, including aims at self-development that have been blocked or frequent fluctuations in a sense of self-identity.

When we describe phenomena, we are already moving toward an explanation of them (Cook 1993). Ingredients of possible explanation are contained in the very words we use for descriptions. For example, we may write down that a person has a pattern of excessive passivity. How this passiveness is described begins to show *when* it occurs, and this provides clues about *why* it occurs. Submissive behaviors may occur more when one patient is with strong, manipulative people. These circumstances may diminish a sense of personal confidence. Another patient may report feeling passive, even paralyzed in action planning, when under fear of abandonment. Subservience may be used to avoid risk of abandonment.

Topics of Concern

Most patients initially identify some topics of concern that are hard for them to resolve on their own. Add these to your list of phenomena. For example, a patient may report a sense of blocked grief for a relative who has been dead for years. A goal of that patient may be to complete mourning, but that aim has been blocked. Examples of other blocked goals include the inability to control rage, to love, to become independent, to take responsibility, to be assertive, to concentrate on work, or to compete.

Systematic Listing of Phenomena

It is not necessary to use a fixed format for listing phenomena. A simple notation will serve for the formulation of most cases. Formulation of complex, difficult, or deeply studied cases (as in training situations) may use systematic formats. Two examples of such systematic formats for listing of phenomena follow.

☐ Case Example: Mrs. Sea

Patricia Sea was married to James Sea. They had children and lived in relative security and happiness. Unexpectedly, James Sea was violently killed. Patricia Sea was shocked. At first she felt numb and depersonalized and merely continued the necessary motions of her life. During the ensuing months, she experienced symptoms of anxiety and depression as well as intrusive images and pangs of emotion about James. More than a year later, she felt frozen in grief. She intuitively knew that her mourning was incomplete and somehow blocked.

Initial interviews explored her current and past experiences. She met criteria for both major depressive disorder and posttraumatic stress disorder. Table 2–1 contains phenomena listed from her evaluation. The format for this table divided phenomena into symptoms, signs, problems of living, and unresolved topics. Table 2–1 is like the problem-oriented record used in medical charts (Weed 1969). The list provides an index for assessing change as time progresses.

Table 2–1.	List of phenomena from the case of Mrs. Sea

Symptoms

Feeling depressed when she "should be happy."[a]

Trouble sleeping, fatigue.

Feeling tense, irritable, and under pressure.

Episodes of socially embarrassing, uncontrolled sobbing.

Intrusive images and nightmares related to fantasies of how husband died.

Pangs of hard-to-describe but negative emotions that felt unbearable if they did not quickly subside.

Signs

Generally articulate, she cuts off topics related to her reactions to her husband's death.

Usually clear but unclear when talking about a new relationship with a man with whom she may become more intimate.

Problems in living

Takes good care of her children, but excessively shields them from knowing about their father's death. For example, did not reveal that there was a grave site. She avoids going there herself, although she thinks she ought to go herself and take her children as well.

Loses her temper and feels bad afterward.

Topics of concern

Uncertain about whether to put the death behind her or to confront the grief she feels she has buried.

Conflicted and indecisive about whether to remain independent or to deepen an attractive new intimacy.

[a]Chief complaint.

Mrs. Sea's chief complaints focused on symptoms of depression. But she also dreaded her tendency to suddenly experience intrusive images of James and her pangs of emotion about his loss. She felt vulnerable to being overwhelmed by such a flood of feelings on any reminder of his death. She avoided such reminders of her loss because she believed her intrusive symptoms would not be worked through to a point of completion of mourning.

☐ Case Example: Mr. Green

Seymour Green, a 42-year-old man, provides a second example of the listing of phenomena as a first step of formulation. He came to psychotherapy with a chief complaint of feeling "anxious and depressed." These feelings had recently flared up because his sister told him she would be leaving the apartment they had shared for 14 years. She was 35 years old and about to marry a man she had been dating for 3 months.

Mr. Green worked at an unusually secure, quiet, and undemanding job. He felt at ease with his sister, and they spent most of their time in their own rooms when at home together. He had dimly expected she would never marry and was startled by her engagement. He had wished to marry, but felt it was impossible. He had courted some women, but found that frustration during erotic overtures led to excessive anger on his part. He then felt anxious, guilty, and overwhelmed with shame.

For years, he had no social activities except for regular religious attendance and work on an antipornography committee stemming from his religious group. He had been deaf since an accident during adolescence, but he did not make contacts in the deaf community, although these had been offered.

After taking a psychiatric history, the therapist made a diagnosis of generalized anxiety disorder and mixed personality disorder with avoidant and narcissistic features. Table 2–2 lists phenomena for Mr. Green. Because Mr. Green actually stated his chief complaint as "anxious and depressed," this phrase is emphasized.

Mr. Green's avoidance of desired courtship situations stood in contrast to his goal of engaging in love, sexual activity, and marrying. Mr. Green greatly feared becoming enraged on sexual frustration and felt guilty when he remembered acting on his hostility. The hostility led to rejections.

Avoiding erotic situations reduced the danger of experiencing rage, guilt, and despair. Mr. Green joined a religious group in an antipornography campaign that involved reviewing and condemning illicit materials. This looking-with-criticism was a kind of substitutive protective behavior. It gained him social contacts, but not the satisfactions he desired, so he still felt lonely.

Biological and Sociological Phenomena

In addition to abnormal psychological phenomena, list abnormal biological and social-context phenomena. They also need explanation

Table 2–2.   List of phenomena from the case of Mr. Green

Symptoms

Anxious and depressed[a]

Feels excessively tense

Dry mouth

Butterflies in stomach

Headaches

Back pain

Partially deaf

Signs

Seems unduly vigilant, wary

Hands tremble

Interest in pornography investigation seems compulsive

Seems low in ordinary "common sense" about people

Avoids discussing his attitude toward his sister's marriage

Does not organize "paragraph" sequences of ideas well although sentences are conceptually clear and grammatically correct

Seems conflicted in his attitudes toward deafness

Cannot hear whispering or a low voice, but understands my ordinary speaking voice

Problems in living

Social isolation

Hard to act confidently

Hard to make friends

Hard to trust others

Topics of concern

Too dependent on sister, hard to arrive at a clear plan of what to do next, but desires marriage

Embarrasses himself and feels guilty about cursing a woman because fears being alone in old age

Hard to feel accepting of himself as he is

---

[a]Chief complaint.

and treatment. Biological inclusions might range from the symptoms of deafness, headaches, back pain, and muscle tremors in Mr. Green to, in other patients, muscle weakness, hormone imbalance, or electrolyte abnormalities. Findings on laboratory tests such as high levels of thyroid-stimulating hormones or low calcium would be inclusions for the list. Similarly, social situations that might be listed as phenomena may range from difficulties in mastery of new responsibilities to episodes of becoming distressed after episodes of stigmatization, harassment, or prejudice.

History of Phenomena

Once we have listed current phenomena, we can describe their historical development as a time sequence. When did a symptom begin and in relation to what events? Were there precipitants? Are there contexts that made it hard to recover from symptoms? Are there relevant phenomena that occurred in the past, but then disappeared? Who in the past had similar symptoms and problems? A time chart by years, months, weeks, and days is a valuable aid when phenomena are complex. Modern computers are useful for organizing information in this way (Stinson and Horowitz 1993).

Linking Clear Selection of Phenomena to Psychotherapy Technique

A careful process of listening, inquiring, and selecting problems leads to activity in therapy. The first interventions are a check on our empathy. We tell patients about their experiences using our words. The patient may respond, and a give-and-take leads to useful clarifications. This kind of discourse helps focus the treatment, and it establishes a strong therapeutic alliance, a sense of working together. Feedback reveals to your patient your expertise, concern, and empathy.

Patients seek expert help for problems that they are unable to solve on their own. They are not sure that the problems can be solved even within a therapeutic alliance. Sometimes they are unsure that the clinician they see is the right kind of expert. Identification by the clinician of relevant dilemmas can give them a sense of hope and trust. They realize the clinician will not dangerously oversimplify hard, vexing conundrums.

The list of phenomena clarifies the aims of treatment. The focus of therapy for Mrs. Sea, at least initially, will be on helping her review her loss in relation to her own potential future identities. She is depressed. Are the warded-off ideas and emotions leading into this state? She cuts off topics about her husband and avoids reminders. What theme is she avoiding? She was a wife; would she ever want to resume that role? The focus of attention in therapy will not be just loss and fear of sadness. It will include who she was, what she lost, who she feels like now, and who she wants to become in the future. The focus presented to Mrs. Sea will view her avoidance of reminders as a defensive stance to be gradually set aside. Her depressive mood will be viewed as a state that may be improved by reducing avoidance, finding out how to mourn safely, and prescribing antidepressant medications if swift progress is not made in psychotherapy.

The focus presented to Mr. Green will concern his beliefs and behavioral tendencies in relation to women and his evaluations of himself. Which of his "stories" reveal patterns of what goes wrong when he is seeing acquaintances? Why has he spurned options of joining the deaf community? When and how does he feel frustrated? What are his beliefs about his relationship with his sister and her new husband? The exploration will aim at a deeper understanding of his capacities and motives, and help him fit them to social options so he feels less anxiety, improves his functions, and thus can become less lonely.

Summary

Selecting the most important phenomena clarifies subsequent tasks that involve the explanation of how and why these phenomena occur and plans on how to alter this causation. Some phenomena may be hidden early; for this reason, we keep lists open ended. The list provides an initial focus for treatment, and it assures the patient that the therapist can understand his or her experiences.

Chapter 3

STATES OF MIND

In our systematic approach to formulation, after we select phenomena, we then look for the states in which symptoms do and do not occur. We are especially alert for states of loss of control over behavior, and we may be able to see if problems relate to motivational conflict by inferring configurations of desired, dreaded, and defensive states.

Formulation of various states of mind is important for three reasons. First, attention to states can clarify variations in symptomatic experiences and maladaptive behaviors. Second, labeling states clarifies emotion and control of emotion in a language a patient can understand. The third reason, especially relevant in personality disorders, is that we can begin to identify cyclical patterns of interpersonal disturbances in relationships.

What Are States of Mind?

A state of mind is a pattern of conscious experiences and interpersonal expressions (Allen 1977; Carr 1983; Docherty et al. 1978; Federn 1952; Horowitz 1979/1987). The elements that combine to form the pattern that is recognized as a state include verbal and nonverbal expressions of ideas and emotions. Typical styles of bodily movement and characteristic qualities of relating to others may vary from state to state.

I find that it helps to start by noticing emotional coloration and the apparent degree of control of emotional expression. We do not look for all possible states of an individual, just a group of important and recurrent ones. I find it useful to consider states in both gener-

31

alized and individualized ways. General categories of states can be used for numerous cases. One can also define individualized states to specify what makes a given case unique.

General State Categories

Four general categories of state description are especially useful, and my colleagues and I have shown they can be reliably identified by independent clinical observers viewing videotapes of patients in psychotherapy (Horowitz et al. 1994b). I call them undermodulated, overmodulated, well-modulated, and shimmering states.

Undermodulated states include impulsive, relatively unregulated displays of feeling and actions that may be explosive, blatant, and raw. They may entail eruptions of usually restrained impulses. Most psychiatric symptoms occur more frequently in undermodulated states. Patients are prone to add anxiety about being out of control to their other problems when they experience such states. Histrionic, narcissistic, antisocial, and borderline personality disorders may present with complaints about an excessive frequency and intensity of such states.

In contrast, patients in *overmodulated* states appear excessively self-restrained or rigid. They may display a poker face, pretend unfelt attitudes, or manifest what looks like a strong indifference to friendly empathy. Many rigid aspects of personality are first reflected in an apparent inability to shift out of overmodulated states and into more spontaneous and vital communications with others. Obsessive-compulsive personality disorders and other typologies lacking in emotional spontaneity may present such states more frequently than others.

Both undermodulated and overmodulated states are deflections from *well-modulated* states. In well-modulated or working states, we observe relatively harmonious accord across modes of expression. The person feels and appears to be in self-command even when expressing intense and distressing emotions and troublesome ideas. A sad mood, for example, could be experienced in well-modulated or undermodulated ways, and this distinction makes a big difference to personal and clinical appraisals about the experiences related to sadness.

Another kind of deflection from well-modulated states can be described as a *shimmering* state. Shimmering states involve rapid oscillations of discrepant behaviors. There may be leakage of emotional expressions alternating rapidly with signs of stifling emotion. Shimmering states may have discords in emotion. For example, feelings expressed in the face may be unlike the emotions proclaimed in words or vocal tone. There may be a quick shuffling between contradictory kinds of expressions verbally and nonverbally.

The states just mentioned—undermodulated, overmodulated, well-modulated, and shimmering—are simple categories. Such terms may help patients in self-observation. Patients may learn to make a useful distinction between their aims to eradicate completely a negative feeling they experience in undermodulated states, and their aims to experience and express their feelings in well-modulated states. For example, a patient prone to tantrums and towering, uncontrolled rages may explicitly or implicitly request that the therapist use techniques that eradicate hostility altogether. The therapist may point out that even were such techniques to exist, the goal is not a useful one. Rather, an aim might be to learn to express anger and frustration early and in a well-regulated and purposive manner.

The important point being made by these four general categories of states is that a given emotion does not always have to be experienced in the same kind of state. A patient who is frequently angry may feel the anger differently and express it quite differently in different states of mind, as illustrated in Table 3–1. A habitually anxious patient may have quite a variety of fearful states, as illustrated in Table 3–2.

Individualized Labels for States

From general categories, we can move to state descriptions individually tailored to the individual patient.

☐ Case Example: Mrs. Sea

Mrs. Sea, whom we met in Chapter 2 and whose husband had died violently (see Table 2–1), felt pangs of emotion and intrusive images about her dead husband most intensely when she was in an *under-*

Table 3–1.   Some angry states of mind showing a gradient from under- to overmodulated states

State label	State description
Undermodulated	
Blind rage	Not thinking, all impulsive expression of hostility; wishes to demolish and destroy other(s) causing frustration to the self; unaware of ever loving or even faintly liking the other(s)
Shimmering	
Sullenness and grudging	Surly and aloof, but irritable; blurts out and then quickly suppresses or disavows anger; easily insulted
Well modulated	
Annoyance	Aware of anger with intended, controlled expressions of irritation; appropriately firm or sharp with other(s) (anger is not overgeneralized nor displaced)
Bantering sarcasm	Able to deliver teasing, good-tempered barbs while remaining aware of affection for current object of hostility and aware that conversation is converting anger to humor
Overmodulated	
"Pro forma"	Feeling numb, although aware of current potential for anger and inhibition of it at an intellectualized level; exhibiting a conspicuously insulated pattern in which actions of the self are rigidly formalized

modulated state individually labeled as intrusive agony of grief. In this state, she experienced sudden waves of unbearable bodily sensation, so strong that she felt she might die. During this state, she would sob in public, and then feel ashamed about losing control before others.

At other times, she felt out of control, or she suffered a paralysis of action in a depleted, apathetic, and uninterested state of mind, a state labeled as dull apathetic depression. She could not dispel it or get out of it, although she wanted to. Another state she disliked be-

Table 3–2.   Some anxious or fearful states of mind, showing a gradient
              from under- to overmodulated states

State label	State description
Undermodulated	
Distraught panic	Feeling of weak knees, lump in throat, dry mouth, faintness, heart pounding or palpitating, flutters or tingles, sweating; feeling like collapsing; inability to focus eyes; ideas of immediately impending harm to self or others; feelings of terror or dread; excessive startle response
Shimmering	
Apprehensive vigilance	Feeling worried about having made or being about to make wrong decisions; having trouble concentrating because of jumbled images; restless body with twitching of eyes; racing thoughts; tense; too alert to outside stimuli; stifling by composing face
Well modulated	
Worry	Feeling afraid; monitoring for signs of possible threats; expressing concerns; seeking information and help; mentally rehearsing possible actions
Overmodulated	
Numbness	Feeling insulated; avoiding threatening ideas or memories; withdrawing

cause it felt out of control was one in which she had a flare of temper and criticized others in a way she then regretted. There were, then, three important and varied undermodulated states in which she felt out of control: intrusive agony of grief, dull apathetic depression, and flare of criticism.

These undermodulated states stood in contrast to *overmodulated states* in which she felt or appeared to others as too controlled. One was a cool and poised state, in which she appeared a bit wooden and felt inside as if she were insulated and remote from connection to the world. She also felt under pressure, a state in which she deliberately and rigidly worked very, very hard. The aim was to be too busy to think about the loss of James, her husband.

In a *shimmering state*, her struggle with grief produced some tendency to lamentation blended with efforts to stifle this and other emotional reactions. She felt tense in social situations because she feared a shift into her intrusive agony of grief.

All these states contrasted with two *well-modulated states*. We called one poignant sorrow, in which she could pine for James and yet not be ashamed or worried about being out of control of her feelings. The other we called happily excited, in which she could feel vibrantly alive and involved in her social, caretaking, and work relationships. These states of mind of Mrs. Sea are summarized in Table 3–3.

As it happens, we can often and usefully formulate a dynamic pattern of several states. We can do so using a configuration that follows the wish-fear-defense model of psychodynamics, as illustrated in Figure 3–1.

Mrs. Sea had a desired state, as shown in Figure 3–2, of being

Table 3–3. States of mind of Mrs. Sea

State label	State description
Undermodulated	Intrusive agony of grief: intrusive images and pangs of emotion, feeling ashamed at losing control before others
	Apathetic depression: depleted feelings, uninterested in everything
	Flare of criticism: too short-tempered with others
Shimmering	Struggle with grief: momentary tearing or glaring with momentary stifling of emotion
Well modulated	Poignant sorrow: feeling sad, pining, and having remembrance of loss without losing control
	Happily excited: engaged vivaciously and productively
Overmodulated	Cool and poised: feeling numb and floating inside, insulated and remote with others
	Pressured: working hard, keeping too busy to think

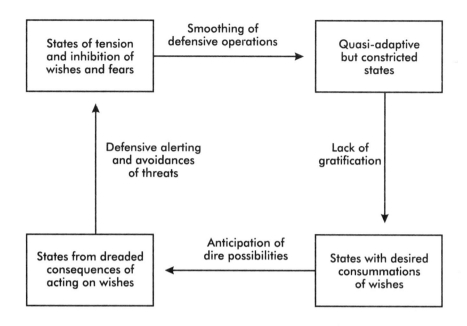

Figure 3-1. Wish-fear dilemmas and defensive compromises. The patient presents symptoms *(upper left)*, makes compromises *(upper right)* between hopes *(lower right)* and fears *(lower left)*.

happily excited and a dreaded state of intrusive agony of grief. The shimmering state of struggle with grief was a problematic compromise. It was less painful than the intrusive agony of grief, but still problematic in that she was embarrassed. When tears welled in her eyes, she dabbed them away quickly, averting her gaze, and shifted topics away from sad ones. As soon as she could stabilize her ideas and feelings, she might shift into the more modulated cool and poised state.

Mrs. Sea was helped by viewing her cool and poised state as a defensive avoidance of her intrusive agony of grief. Her relationship with her therapist helped her maintain a middle ground, a state like poignant sorrow in which she could remember and lament without feeling out of control. Work accomplished during this state reduced the frequency of dull apathetic depression and flares of criticism targeted at loved ones. By becoming aware of these changes in frequency, she saw an early sign of progress and gained hope for a good outcome

Problematic compromise	Quasi-adaptive compromise
• Struggle with grief	• Cool and poised
• Agony of grief	• Happily excited
Dreaded	**Desired**

Figure 3–2.   Configuration of states for Mrs. Sea.

from therapy. That, in turn, increased her motivation for work in treatment and improved her trusting relationship with her therapist.

Cycles of States

Some DSM-IV (American Psychiatric Association 1994) Axis I symptom disorders go through phases in which sets of symptoms vary. Posttraumatic stress disorder is a common example. Some Axis II personality disorders manifest themselves almost specifically as cycles of states. Patterns of forming and breaking up intimate relationships and work arrangements occur.

☐ Case Example: Mr. Keith

Mr. Keith, in well-modulated states, was competent, intelligent, and highly skilled in computer programming. He was in high demand at his corporation, but he had a recurrent pattern of regression and progression. Sometimes his behavioral pattern was frantic, unstable, self-mutilating, and irrational. He had received a diagnosis of borderline personality disorder.

Each cycle into an unstable, violent, and extremely irrational state began with overmodulated states in which he displayed obsessional thinking and compulsive and conspicuously slow body movements. He would become concerned at being abandoned by someone. Then he had shimmering states of fear, disavowal of concerns about abandonment, and hypochondriacal preoccupations that led to demands for medical attention. These states seemed defensive against what

Problematic compromise	Quasi-adaptive compromise
• Hypochondriacal	• Obsessional and slow
• Terror-stricken	• Competently working
Dreaded	**Desired**

Figure 3–3. Configuration of states for Mr. Keith.

then followed, a state of irrational panic in which he experienced delusional ideas about people trying to harm him and unbidden images of bodily fragmentation. The fragmentation of his body was presumably caused by the malicious intentions of evil others. From this state, he shifted to one of sheer terror that he, strangely, could relieve by inflicting bodily injury on himself, such as slicing through the skin of his forearm with a razor. He then felt a soothing release of tension and received emergency room help to suture his wound.

On recovering from his irrational states, Mr. Keith transiently repeated his overmodulated compulsive and obsessing state, then returned to his well-modulated and competently working states. Figure 3–3 and Figure 3–4 provide such a configuration and cycle.

Understanding Contradictions

Contradictory behaviors may occur in different states. The overall pattern may be seen in a cycle of states. For example, a patient with a histrionic personality disorder may begin a cycle in a theatrically self-dramatizing state of apparent sexuality to attract attention. After that, the patient may feel rejected and may show volatile hostility. Next, the patient may shift to a depressed state of suicidal rumination. This may be followed by a state of sympathy-provoking plaintiveness, as a way to seek caregiving and protective behaviors from the therapist. Then a repetition of sexualized self-dramatization to gain desired attention from others may renew the cycle.

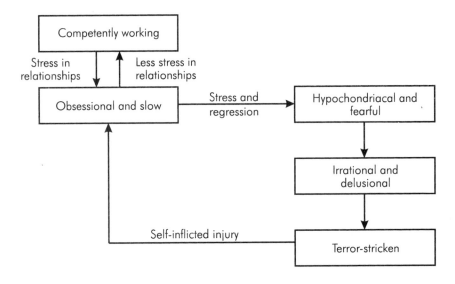

Figure 3–4.   Cycle of states for Mr. Keith.

Recognizing repeated state cycles promotes understanding. A patient may learn to predict what could happen. Forewarned is forearmed; the patient may gain better mastery over potential repetitions. Histrionic patients may learn to slow down and think before acting. They may learn to examine the motives of other people rather than see them as projections, and may learn how to reduce self-dramatization and increase authenticity to attract others who are not so likely to exploit them. Routes to slower affiliations may be explored. As a result, the patient may establish interpersonal relationships that are less likely to rupture. More stable relationships will, in turn, protect the patient from plummeting into a dysphoric, suicidal state.

Understanding Triggers That Cause a Shift in State

A state of mind can be triggered by a psychological reminder of a topic of concern, by some biological shift, by an alteration in the current social context, or by a combination of such events. A state transition can be triggered by an internal change in intentions, a review of memory, or the progressing ideas in a fantasy. In addition, a shift in state of mind can be caused by shifts in the play of defensive control processes on the activities of thought and the organizers that affect thought. A change in identity concepts or in relationship conceptualizations can alter state. Formulation seeks to define these reasons for the repetitive shifts from one state to another, and perhaps cycles that combine several types of repetitions.

I have argued so far that describing a state gives us a way of binding various phenomena into a coherent pattern of co-occurrences. Describing several characteristic states of a patient gives us a way of saying how such patterns fluctuate. For example, a coppery and dry mouth, weakness in the knees, a sense of impending catastrophe, butterflies in the stomach, and urgent clinging to or seeking a companion may co-occur in an undermodulated state of near panic. Calling the state "near panic" may serve to label the combination and distinguish the state from another one of well-modulated fear in which there is reflective contemplation of how to plan for possibly impending catastrophe without the features of near panic just mentioned. This makes it sound like phenomena are "smaller than" a state. Because phenomena are contained within an overall state, this is, indeed, an accurate appraisal.

We can also understand, however, how a single phenomenon might trigger the occurrence of other, associated phenomena. The catalyst might shift the individual into a state of mind in which these phenomena occur together. With this line of cause and effect, it may seem that some symptomatic phenomena are "bigger" than the state as a concept. For example, a person might have a tendency to irregular heartbeats for reasons of cardiac anatomy and physiology (e.g., mitral valve prolapse syndrome). On feeling a thump in the chest, there might be associated ideas to heart attacks and death: the person might then experience the near-panic state with its general pattern of features including a sense of dying as an impending catastrophe, weakness in the knees, butterflies in the stomach, and so forth. So it may be important not to let "bigger than" and "smaller than" issues cloud the steps of formulation in which phenomena are related to states. It is generally useful to proceed in the order given, to define first phenomena and then states that contain phenomena.

Utilizing State Formulations
in Psychotherapy

One advantage of this system of formulation is that its language can be used with patients, not just professionals. Having some labels by which to recognize a state or even an impending state transition gives the patient a sense of heightened control over thought and behavior. A phrase such as "agony of grief" or "flare of criticism" may be derived from the patient's own terms. After the patient and therapist arrive at full descriptions, the allied pair can use the label as a shorthand term to refer to the fuller description.

Some states have qualities of attraction and repulsion that can be useful in considering the goals of the patient. Naming desired states, such as happily excited, clarifies a patient's goals and his or her dilemma in achieving them. Achieving desired states can be discussed as a step-by-step process. Suppose a patient with a work block wants to be a great author. The state of triumph the patient will feel on winning a great literary prize is in the remote and not necessarily plausible future. But the patient might achieve a state of concentration while writing paragraphs now. The patient can attend to the difference between being in a state of hard work, concentrating on writing a good sentence, and being in a state of indifferent word shuffling and diddling. Awareness of being in a "diddling state" can lead to an intention to shift into a productive, working state, choosing what actions to stop and what actions to take.

During therapy, we can help patients avoid repeating hazardous state cycles that can lead to maladaptive outcomes. Control may be easier for the patient to achieve earlier in a state cycle rather than later. The triggers that evoke dreaded states can be identified. Attention can lead to the preparation of alternative routes of response. When the triggers occur, they are less startling, and sudden state shifts are less likely to occur. The patient learns to become alert to "early warning signs" and learns how to make early "steer clear" efforts.

After state stabilization, we may consider and interpret to the patient possible configurations of desired, dreaded, and defensive compromise states. Unwanted states and moods, once labeled, can be examined in four temporal spaces: current outside situations, the here and now of the therapy situation, memories and fantasies from the past, and imagined states of the future.

Looking at the development of a state may be useful. For example, understanding identification through mimicry of a state witnessed in a parent may increase a sense of how to change. A patient may complain of loss of control over his impulses to react with hostility when his children are disobedient. His most dreaded state may be one of towering and impulsive rage. Once the patient and therapist have clarified the rage states, the therapist can ask *when* they started, *how* they evolved, and *who* may have exhibited such rages in the past. The rage state may have been experienced from a parent who abused the patient. Recognition of learning by identification may increase reflective self-control of the current problematic states.

Social contexts are also pertinent. Some cultures sanction corporal punishment and encourage children to strict obedience; others do not. Biological factors are pertinent as well. Loss of control over violent impulses might be more frequent if exposure to a chemical used at work reduced brain regulatory capacities, or if there was alcoholic bingeing or some other substance abuse. Biopsychosocial formulations will be necessary for a complete approach.

States of the Therapist

Patients come to learn our states as therapists as well as vice versa. Sometimes our own states may usefully enter into formulations of current issues. For example, a therapist in the midst of his or her own mourning process may cry more readily when a patient brings up issues of loss. It may be valuable to acknowledge such events by identifying your own personal states.

At other times, it may be useful for us to make "we"-type identifications of states. These identify the state of the therapeutic pair or of a small therapy group. Examples include saying, "We are in a jumbled or foggy state right now, but we usually work ourselves out of it into more clarity about what is going on," or "We are not together in a working state right now. I am not sure why that is; do you have any ideas?" Or, after a long silence in which the patient seems to be "at work" rather than "resisting," but now seems worried at being silent, the therapist may support the patient by saying, "Useful things can go on when we just sit quietly together without talking."

State-Oriented Technique

Treatment can be usefully state oriented. Different techniques are appropriate in different states. Helping the patient to increase control and gain state stability is a top priority when a patient presents risks to self and others in undermodulated states. Increasing a sense of safety and reducing resistance to emotional expression is a high priority in patients who present only overmodulated states.

A useful example of how treatment may be state oriented is found in considering the phases of states found in stress response syndromes, such as posttraumatic stress disorders and in crisis reactions or adjustment disorders (Horowitz 1973, 1976, 1986).

After an initial outcry phase, we may find that stress response moves toward such a global increase of control over emotionality that overmodulated states of denial and numbing are stabilized. Later, phases marked by undermodulated states may then occur, as manifested by intrusions such as unbidden images, unwanted recollections, and pangs of emotion. Techniques during the intrusive states are different from those used in denial states.

During outcry or intrusion phases, the first aim of treatment is social, biological, and psychological state stabilization. Our goal is to reduce the frequency of problematic and dreaded undermodulated states that contain many symptoms and demoralize the patient. The next goal is to deal with current problems and unresolved memories, such as incompletely assessed and integrated stressor life events. A third goal is to integrate a sense of identity past, present, and future. This goal can be addressed with some success after reaching the first two goals.

The best progress is likely to be made in a well-modulated working state with some oscillations into shimmering states as powerful issues are confronted. In brief therapy, and in general, the goal is to deal with passions, emotions, motives, memories, and fantasies in states in which conscious reflection is at its most rational, and when new choices and plans can be made and remembered. State-oriented technique aims first at stabilizing rational, working states in which the patients are neither overmodulated nor undermodulated in expressing authentic ideas and feelings. In long-term, exploratory, and self-developmental psychotherapies, after a strong therapeutic alliance is established, incursions into undermodulated states may be useful.

Stabilizing Well-Modulated Working States

Well-modulated states can be stabilized in a safe therapy context. The most important thing we do to establish that context is to emphasize the characteristics of a therapeutic alliance, as is discussed in greater detail in a later chapter on views of self and other. Pacing is also important: there should be enough concern for problems to keep the process moving, but not so much confrontation with self-impairing issues as to flood the patient with emotion.

I think that clarifying current and future dilemmas of choice is more important than identifying problem-causing choices that have been made in the past. Both, however, are important. Empathic understanding is conveyed as we clarify why the patient has been caught up in problems that he or she has not been able to solve before without expert help. In the future, we can offer patients new ways to avoid the obstacles to solutions and the various dead ends or traps than have ensnared and entangled them in the past. This empathy builds a sense of joint work on solvable problems, restoring morale and stabilizing working states of frank discourse.

Techniques When a Patient Has Entered or Is About to Enter an Undermodulated State

When the patient is in an undermodulated state, we may encourage restraint from actions such as substance abuse or binge eating that seem to provide immediate relief but actually risk harm. We reinforce the adaptive value of planning in advance. We help the patient to rehearse plans such as "thinking before acting." We help the patient bolster working states of mind in which emotional topics can be examined in a well-modulated manner.

We model such routes of contemplation by speaking clearly, slowly, and calmly while naming the ideas and emotions that have flooded the patient. We also help the patient slow down ideation to avoid emotional flooding. We repeat frequently and organize the sequence of expressions. We deal with the implications of difficult topics one step at a time, allowing time for recovery of emotional equilibrium before going on to the next step. (Sometimes the review of preceding steps is calming, but in some patients it can have the opposite effect.)

During or near undermodulated states, we are generally well advised to help the patient regain organization and control of emotion by slowing down the rate of expression of arousing ideas, memories, and fantasies. If we talk slowly and calmly, in a way that repeats what the patient has said, we may accomplish this aim. Such repetitions can add ideational structure. They often give the patient a chance to listen and reflect. Our talk also indicates to the patient our acceptance of his or her communications. We speak in a well-modulated state what the patient has expressed in an undermodulated state, and this model changes some aspects of meaning. Silence also can be very useful, permitting the patient a period of restoration.

Interpretations of the meaning of nonverbal behavior and of defensive avoidances and layering are not likely to be clearly processed by a patient in a state of information overload. These interpretations are best used in well-modulated states, not undermodulated ones.

Techniques When the Patient Has Entered or Is About to Enter a Shimmering State

Empathic listening is especially important during shimmering states of mind. As the patient struggles with conflicting motives and meanings, it may be useful to make very brief repetitions of whatever the patient has said and then stifled. Then, in the expert activity loop discussed in Chapter 1 (see again Figure 1–1), you may interpret both the expressed contents and why these are hard to contemplate.

I think you may also find it useful to label discordant emotions with aptly chosen words. Because the patient is usually experiencing complex medleys of emotions, such clarification is not easy. It may be useful to say so. You might say something like, "I think it is hard for you to say all you are feeling because you experience such a simultaneous mix of shame for skipping class, anger at the professor who might criticize you too much, and fear for what will happen because you missed the test."

We had a group of judges score each half-minute of video-recorded psychotherapy sessions for the predominant state of the patient; they were reliable in their independent judgments. The states they scored as undermodulated or shimmering states more frequently contained unresolved topics (Horowitz et al. 1993c, 1994c). This study indicates empirically why it is important to observe what topics go with what states and to use entry into a shimmering state as a sign of what topics are most conflictual. Then the therapist can concentrate on understanding those topics.

Techniques When the Patient Has Entered or Is About to Enter an Overmodulated State

We need not intervene if the patient has shifted into an overmodulated state just as a temporary respite from a period of high emotional intensity. Once equilibrium is restored, the patient will change back to a working state. In other situations, we may encourage the patient toward the less rigid use of defensive control processes. We may say whatever we can authentically to increase a sense of trust in our openness to listening to troubles and the safety that can be found in therapy.

We may want to encourage authentic expression as a way to get attention, rather than feigning states that feel unauthentic. We will usually not respond to behavioral provocations to shift into social "chit-chat." We will instead interpret the defensive purposes of shifting into any state displaying pretended emotions or into states inappropriate. In doing so, we will also compassionately label feelings that are *like* those feigned and that can be felt *authentically* in other states.

Further techniques involve interpreting how, when, and why the patient may fear entry into dreaded state of mind. This may include interpretation of ideas and feelings that are warded off. We can identify defensive control processes and counter them. That is why defensive control processes are considered in the next chapter.

Integrating Psychotherapy, Pharmacotherapy, and Social Interventions

Medication or social supports may be prescribed when psychological interventions are inadequate to reduce prolonged undermodulated states of confusion, terror, desperate action, or depression. A companion may prevent some panic attacks, or sleeping with parents may help a frightened child to get needed rest. Antianxiety, antidepressant, or antipsychotic medications may reduce protracted undermodulated states of fear, inertia, or delusionality, respectively.

Once a state has stabilized, attention can be directed to what causes these states. It may be unwise, however, to focus on upsetting memories and fantasies or to use reverie-inducing psychotherapy techniques, such as free association to problematic foci, before undermodulated states are reduced in frequency and intensity.

Summary

State analysis reduces phenomena into useful packages. It clarifies when symptoms appear and dissipate. Many interpersonal problems can be clarified as cycles of states.

Attention in psychotherapy may be directed toward stabilizing working states. As we come to know a patient, we gain an intuitive sense of impending state transitions. Anticipating undermodulated states, we can slow down the rate of information processing without derailing discourse. Anticipating overmodulated states, we can intervene to reduce resistance by showing the patient that therapy is safer than imagined. During shimmering states, we can concentrate on clarifications of both what is being expressed and what is warded off, and why there is conflict over disclosure.

Chapter 4

TOPICS OF CONCERN AND DEFENSIVE CONTROL PROCESSES

In our next step, we can further clarify topics of concern that we infer may play a part in symptom formation. Because patients often defensively avoid topics that, when considered, might lead them into dreaded and undermodulated states of mind, this task is not easy. It is important, however, because by taking this step we move closer to establishing a focus for treatment. By identifying obstacles to clarity, we move closer to targeting resistances to counteract during treatment.

Psychotherapy, by its basic ground rules, fosters clarity. State analysis prepares the way for deeper observations on topics of concern and excessively avoidant defenses. Shifts away from well-modulated states may occur when conflictual topics are broached, as we have shown in empirical and quantitative research on personal meanings (Horowitz et al. 1994b, 1994c, 1995c). Some shifts in state occur for clearly defensive reasons, as ways to avoid more dreaded states of mind. In addition, some symptoms occur in states that seem to be caused by particular social circumstances, ones that indicate psychological topics of concern. For example, a man whose chief complaint was binge drinking told me he got drunk after not receiving an expected present from a family member, went on a binge when a friend asked him to stop calling, and got drunk when not invited to join a group of co-workers for a party. That made it clear that a topic of concern might involve a theme of rejection.

The initially emergent clarity of important psychological themes will vary in different types of cases. In crisis-induced depressions, adjustment disorders, phobic responses to frights, and posttraumatic stress disorders, life change events are clear topics of concern. How the self interprets and responds to the altered situation is a relevant question. In contrast, depressions presenting as vegetative symptoms of loss of enjoyment in life, sexual disinterest, sleep disturbance, and weight loss may not yield clear psychological themes until, after many interviews, repetitive conflict, unintegrated memories, or persisting irrational beliefs about the future despite mood elevation became clear foci for attention. An exaggerated degradation of the self and a dysfunctional pessimism might be present early but disappear as mood elevation occurred. The latter topical concerns may have been, in part, based on biologically based state shifts.

Close observation of displays, even very brief displays of emotion, may identify some themes of importance. Pangs of emotion are especially important to observe. The sudden surge of feeling may be expressed for less than a second, but may flag the relevance of a concurrently spoken idea or an incipient inferred, unexpressed idea. The quality of intrusiveness of ideas themselves is also important. Some topics of concern are identified because a patient says "I just keep on thinking about this . . ." Other patients will say clearly what they do not know how to think through: "I don't know how to decide . . .," "Tell me what to do about . . .," "It is hopeless to realize that. . . ."

Finding Obscured Ideas in Topics of Concern

A topic of concern is like an iceberg. Some ideas and feelings are on the surface; other themes float beneath the surface, bob up now and again, but are usually obscure. A bit of detective work to find these ideas and feelings may be indicated. We then can infer *what* is warded off from conscious clarity, *why* it is warded off, and *how* it is obscured (Freud 1926). Such inferences then are related to practical issues of technique—when to encourage expression and why to support defensive coping by avoiding dreaded states of mind.

We have found that very expressive and evocative techniques may be associated with poor outcome of psychotherapy in patients with vulnerabilities to loss of coherence of self-conceptualization. Topics of concern, if fully expressed, may lead to disorganizing strong negative emotions such as anger (Horowitz, Marmar, Weiss, et al. 1984b). Yet, such techniques may be associated with better psychotherapy outcomes in patients who can tolerate anxiety and, sometimes, shame states that occur on expression of usually warded-off elements in topics of concern. That is why the inferences at this step need to be coupled with inferences at the next step of formulation before arriving at a set of techniques for treatment.

Shimmering States of Mind as Special Episodes for Close Observation

Shimmering states of mind were defined in the last chapter. As mentioned, we found quantitative evidence that conflictual and unresolved themes were more frequently expressed during shimmering states (Horowitz et al. 1993c, 1994a, 1994b). What is interesting about this is that shimmering states are ones in which obscure ideas and feelings in topics of concern are both partially expressed and partially stifled. In a safe situation, as can be provided by expert formulation and treatment planning with a good therapeutic alliance, these ideas and feelings can be progressively expressed with less avoidance and distortion.

Some of the nonverbal signs of defensiveness we found most useful in noticing when shimmering states were present included increased frequency and intensity of averting gaze, shielding the face, squirming, jiggling limbs, massaging hands, and closing in the body with tight-limbed postures. Verbal signs of shimmering states included taking back what was just said, minimizing affect by saying phrases like "well, just a little bit," trailing off prematurely by saying "I don't know," or just quitting the topic. We have found clinical observers can reliably identify such signs of dyselaboration (Horowitz et al. 1993a). On observing such signs, you can ask yourself to note the ideas and flickering expressions of emotion that are "nearby" to the shift in state. Then you can consider a very important issue that will help you decide whether to try to foster expression and to increase clarity about these ideas. How irrational is the patient in terms of how they go about avoiding the ideas? If the person is quite irrational in defensive constructions, he or she may be vulnerable to going from shimmering into excessively undermodulated states. Going through defenses may be too threatening to coherence of self-organization.

One may observe signs of defensive control processes and not know what lies beneath the obscuring presentations. That is why this step of formulation is followed by another step, a layering approach to core beliefs about self and others. We get into that in the next chapter. Here we need only consider more carefully how to formulate why and how the person prevents expression of difficult themes.

To repeat: the more irrational the defensiveness—that is, the more distorted the beliefs—the more we must assume our patient is in danger of emotional flooding or entry into dreaded states of mind. We should be very cautious in our exploration of avoided themes and not plunge ahead to seek insight at all costs. Otherwise, exposing a warded-off theme can lead to impulsive behavior, regression into more symptoms, and a profound sense of loss of identity structure. Formulation of expressed and warded-off themes is important, but it need not lead to immediate counterdefensive techniques. We will usually discover that our patient has reasons for obscuring frank discourse.

Motivation for Warding Off Problematic Themes by Use of Defensive Control Processes

Among the most overwhelming or unpleasant human experiences are undermodulated states: mortal terror, darkest despair, towering hostility, and searing shame and guilt. A shift into states that avoid such experiences is accomplished by defensive control processes. Achievement of relative safety carries a cost, which is usually a blunting or blurring of ideas and feelings that might otherwise be confronted directly and rationally.

Patients purchase emotional equilibrium at the price of inadequate chances to prepare for stress and learn from it. For example, prolonged denial of the implications of bad news from a stressor life event may be associated with a feeling of numbness rather than fright, but it does not prepare one for optimum coping with the crisis. A period of denial and numbing may be useful and normal in a first response to a trauma, but it becomes a pathological symptom if it leads to failures to act.

Consider a patient with gangrene who has to give signed consent for a surgical amputation if his or her life is to be saved. The patient may deny the news, provided by the surgeon who asks for the signature, that gangrene leads to septicemia, shock, coma, and eventually death. The aim is to avoid a dreaded state of fear and the horror of feeling worthless and helpless without the limb. Information that might be useful to the patient's survival is not interpreted with its real importance. A psychotherapist might have to intervene rapidly to counteract such denial before septicemia occurs. In our patients' interest, we seek to formulate both the degree to which defenses are useful *and* the degree to which they pose a danger to adaptive functioning.

A patient may habitually inhibit attention to bad news that threatens his or her sense of self-identity. The patient may display a pattern of disavowing actions that repeatedly cause personal impairment. We may need to differentiate current, stress-induced regressions from habitual defensive styles. That kind of differentiation—is the defensiveness current or is it both current and also habitually automatic—may take time. We may make such inferences only through the additive and gradual process of reformulation. It is helpful to remember that some signs of defensive control are due to stressed states and do not necessarily reflect habitual defensive traits of character.

What to Observe to Formulate Defensive Control Processes

As mentioned, abandoning an important, unclearly resolved topic before an apt point of closure is one of our best signs of defensive control processes. Any shifts from our patient's usual manner of communication may also catch our attention. An increase in ideas that are jumbled, started and stopped, or excessively general rather than self-focused may indicate defensiveness. Discords and contradictions between and within verbal and nonverbal communication of emotion are also important. A person may talk clearly and harmoniously about many topics, but shift into stuttering, obscurity, and disjointed ideas when a specific topic is broached. This pattern might indicate the importance of that topic. Once we clearly identify signs of defensiveness, we can look at when they are repeated. In this way, we gradually observe how signs link to certain topics and core themes.

Although we still might not know why a topic was important, we can make a note of it and plan whether to, where to, and how to alter the patient's use of defensive control processes.

Important themes and defensive control processes can also be inferred from stories told about what happens outside the clinical session. A patient who initially came because she abused her child may describe a work failure and then report that when she returned home she had angrily disparaged her child as stupid and inept for breaking a dish. She had placed blame and disgust away from herself. Using role reversal as a defense might be described as shifting from a view of the self as inept to viewing the child as inept. Fault is attributed to the child—the child is to blame and not the self—and hostility is displaced. Warding off a dreaded state of self-disgust by displacing hostility onto a child, leading to a symptom of child abuse, is a partial formulation based on stories like this.

Types of Defensive Control Processes

Clinicians seeing the same videotape of a session with a patient may agree on the manifestations of specific defense mechanisms (Vaillant 1993). In cognitive-behavioral schools of practice, the theoretical construct of defense is seldom specified, although some do regard defenses as important (Young 1990), and obstacles to therapy are considered in such formulations (Persons 1992, 1993). To integrate dynamic and cognitive-behavioral concepts, my colleagues and I have developed a direct observational approach (Horowitz 1986; Horowitz et al. 1992, 1995a). It represents a convergence of psychodynamic theory with modern cognitive science (Horowitz 1988a, 1988b; Horowitz et al. 1990). The result is a simplified tool for observing signs of defensive control processes—a listing of categories of mental activities that can alter emotion (Horowitz and Stinson 1994, 1995).

The list of control processes that affect the contents of themes and topics one may think about and communicate is found in Table 4–1. You can, in psychotherapy, act in ways to counteract each of these defensive maneuvers. That is why formulation of what the patient does repeatedly is valuable.

In general, the defensive control processes that involve *content* (inhibiting attention to topics, concepts, and meanings) form the phenomena of repression, suppression, disavowal, denial, and rationalization. The control processes that involve *form* (mode, time, linkage, arousal) form the phenomena of regression, autistic fantasy, generalization, isolation, and withdrawal. The control processes that can *shift roles of identity* in relation to others can form defenses called projection, projective identification, splitting, dissociation, reaction formation, role reversal, and undoing. Fuller discussions of defense mechanisms are provided elsewhere (Conte and Plutchik 1994; Horowitz 1988a; Horowitz et al. 1995a; J. C. Perry and Cooper 1989; Singer 1990; Vaillant 1992; Zeidner and Endler 1995).

One of the co-determinations of symptom formation may stem from defensive motives. A patient may use a set of defensive operations to ward off impulses, memories, or associations dreaded even more than the symptoms. For example, a patient presenting with anxiety symptoms may need treatment that not only can reduce tension, apprehensiveness, and inhibitions of action, but also alter impulses of self-destruction, rage attacks on others, or acts that will dissolve valuable marital and work contracts.

Consider a suicidally depressed patient as another example. Our first goal will probably be state stabilization with a combination of medications, milieu, and supportive psychotherapy. Once the patient is less likely to enter states of uncontrollable despair, we may find it advisable to deal with the situational and belief-based sources of the degraded self-concepts, sense of abandonment, and dismal expectations of failure in the future. Such midtherapy plans may involve our work with the patient to counteract defensive impediments to frank expression of active but quite irrational beliefs about personal incompetence, worthlessness, and pessimism. Modification of these dysfunctional beliefs may be a key to reducing the likelihood of relapse.

Table 4–1.   Defensive control processes

Content

Shifting attention: Avoids conscious thought, discourse, or action on important unresolved topics by shifting attention to another topic; the shifts may be deliberate (suppression) or may involve less conscious automatic choices (repression, dissociation, disavowal, or denial).

Juggling concepts about a topic: Shifts too often among ideas or emotional valences of ideas, thus preventing a potentially affect-related deepening train of thought; irrelevant details may be amplified. Vital links between ideas and feelings, and between cause and effect, may be obscured.

Sliding meanings and values: Adjusts conceptual weighting by minimizing or exaggerating intentions or emotional salience; the resulting appraisal errors and rationalizations may preserve self-esteem or reduce affect ("sweet lemons" or "sour grapes").

Premature disengaging from topics: Declares important topics or actions "finished" before reaching closure despite awareness of unresolved dilemmas and contradictions, effectively blocking potentially emotional review of important memories or anticipation of likely future events (e.g., interpersonal tensions).

Form

Blocking apt modes of representation: Ineffectively represents ideas and feelings about a topic, engaging either in verbal intellectualizations or in preoccupying fantasies. Both can lead to failure to engage in effective action planning. Discourse may lack imagery, metaphors, and clarity, or else may be excessively metaphoric with poor translation of visual images into clear, concrete, meaningful ideas. Both can reduce reactive emotions.

Shifting time span: Shifts from most pertinent to alternative less relevant temporal contexts (e.g., distant past, recent past, here-and-now, immediate future, distant future) in a manner that avoids or reduces emotionality (e.g., shifts to past memories apparently to avoid confrontation with current relationship difficulties or future jeopardy).

Using poor ideational linkage strategies: Employs intellectualized analysis of generalities when reflective contemplation or recollection of personalized issues and emotional memories is more appropriate; conversely, may use creatively wide-ranging associations when careful adaptive planning is more appropriate. The results may be isolated from identity and emotional responses.

(continued)

Table 4–1.   Defensive control processes *(continued)*

Form *(continued)*

Engaging inappropriate arousal levels: Shifts to an inappropriate level of arousal specifically when addressing a problematic topic; becomes dull, listless, or sleepy or else becomes too excited to do effective contemplation.

Person schemas

Shifting self/other roles: Abruptly shifts to alternate views of self and other or switches attributes of self and others (e.g., projection, role reversal, displacement, compensatory grandiosity), avoiding dreaded states of fear, shame, rage, and guilt.

Rigidly stabilizing compromise roles: Rigidly assumes compromise roles and views of self and other, apparently avoiding desired ones that may have associations with dreaded ones (e.g., wish-fear dilemmas); consequences include avoiding threatening situations and dysphoric emotion, but also include withdrawal, numbing, excessive self-preoccupations, and lack of satisfaction.

Altering valuation schemas: Shifts to an alternate set of values for appraising self or other with idealizing or devaluing consequences (e.g., unrealistically attributing blame to another, unrealistically criticizing oneself).

To clarify these concepts, we now reconsider a case in brief time-limited treatment for a DSM-IV (American Psychiatric Association 1994) Axis I symptom disorder.

☐ Case Example: Mrs. Sea

You will recall Mrs. Sea's prolonged and complicated grief reaction diagnosed as both major depressive disorder and posttraumatic stress disorder. Her anticipations of dreaded, overwhelming states of emotion motivated her to use high levels of defensive control. Her control processes stabilized compromise states in which she avoided themes related to being a wife, either in remembering her dead husband or in envisioning remarriage to a new husband.

More than a year after her traumatic loss, she had recently decided to date men once again. After several awkward attempts, she had developed a rewarding and intimate relationship with Sidney (again, all names are fictitious). However, when she was with Sidney, she had intrusive images of James, her dead husband, as still alive.

She also felt angry at being pressed for more commitment by Sidney. She felt that she was cheating Sidney out of a promising future together, but she felt she was being disloyal to James by finding intimacy with Sidney. These were themes of conflict, and her discourse on them was associated with heightened signs of defensive control processes.

To ward off undermodulated states of intrusive agony of grief, which might occur during intimacy with Sidney, and irritable states marked by flares of criticism directed at Sidney, she used a variety of processes to stabilize her cool, poised compromise state. She inhibited attention to the topics of James' death and her possible marriage to Sidney ("shifting attention" in Table 4–1). She engaged her attention on many work-related topics, even to the extent of piling enormous time demands on herself.

If her attention was directed to the conflictual themes during therapy or during an outside activity by reminders of James or Sidney, she touched on the threatening topic only briefly and then quickly concluded it as "done" ("premature disengaging from topics" in Table 4–1).

She focused on the immediate, near future ("shifting time span" in Table 4–1). Everything with James was past, and she did not consider that past time frame. Everything with Sidney was far in the future, and she also did not consider that time frame. If held to the topic by reminders, she shifted into an overmodulated and remote state and retracted or obscured any expressed emotional attitudes.

One way she could avoid emotion was to ignore thinking of herself as a vibrant woman, interested in a male-female relationship. She instead focused on concepts of herself as a businesswoman, autonomous and independent, and concentrated on improving her effectiveness at work ("shifting self/other roles" and "rigidly stabilizing compromise roles" in Table 4–1).

Mrs. Sea's defensive control processes (observed in interviews) that interfered with mourning are summarized in Table 4–2. She could not reach a relatively completed view of her story of marriage with James—accepting and integrating her memories and feelings, her ups and downs, his good and bad features, and their moments of love and resentment. In particular, she had not yet formed a new belief structure of James as "safely dead"—that is, not suffering, not sentient,

---

Table 4–2.   Defensive control processes of Mrs. Sea

- Inhibits attention to active memories about James (past) and Sidney (future).
- Concentrates attention on present and near-future tasks not involving intimacy.
- Interrupts emotional topics by declarations of "it's over with."
- Retracts or obscures lexical communications that lead toward the emotional heart of topics.
- Inhibits self-schemas as *vibrant woman* and facilitates as a substitute a self-schema as *stoic, independent (unloving) woman.*

---

not haunting her, and not accusing her of cheating on him by being with Sidney. Even were she to view James as sentient, in heaven, knowing of her relationship to James, she did not believe that he would authorize her recovery and continuation with life. Her interruptions of thought meant that, long after James' death, she had not reached a stable state of established beliefs that were in accord with her real situation.

In defense mechanisms terminology, she tended to use *suppression* under stress. Under more severe strain, the inhibition was unconscious rather than consciously chosen; the results were *repressive* rather than suppressive phenomena. She supplemented suppression and repression with *disavowal, denial,* and selective interpersonal *withdrawal.*

☐ Case Example: Mr. Beam

Let us now consider a single episode of observation.

Mr. Beam, a man in his mid-30s, came to treatment for symptoms of anxiety, states of intense doubt about his life choices, and intrusive images of his brother 5 years after his brother had committed suicide. Past history included a childhood injury that left him with a slight but visible physical handicap. He subsequently channeled his energies into intellectual activity. Mr. Beam was successful in his work, but he suffered frequent anxiety over the possibilities of failure. He felt uncertain about making a commitment with women, and he had various approach-avoidance dilemmas that interfered with any long-term relationship.

Mr. Beam's intrusive images of his brother were accompanied by waves of sadness, longing, and restorative ideas that his brother was alive and about to visit him. He imagined his brother entering his room, still alive. He conspicuously avoided disclosing even to close friends that his brother had died, and he was anxious that this serious omission of information would be revealed to them.

After an initial period in psychotherapy, in which Mr. Beam emphasized the importance of his brother's death, he shifted to discussing problems with women and his work, disavowing the relevance of the death. He depreciated the therapist's efforts to focus on the possibility of an incomplete mourning response. He denied active conflicts about his relationship with his brother, but he then experienced an intrusive image of himself at age 5. He wondered why this memory occurred at this time.

In the unbidden image, he saw himself falling down and being scolded by his father in an angry voice. His father felt embarrassed at having a handicapped son, and he was selfish rather than caring. Mr. Beam believed that his father ought to have been more helpful. The "falling" image emerged when he was confronted by the therapist with the possible importance of his brother's death. His brother had "fallen down" in death. Was he avoiding this topic to avoid his remorse over not helping his brother "up" from suicide?

Mr. Beam shifted attention away from an important unresolved topic: his relationship with his brother and his appraisal of the meaning of his brother's suicide. If it did become a focus, he inhibited thoughts that his concentration on his own work kept him from helping his brother and encouraged thoughts that *he* was not helped because the suicide interfered with his work. That concept allowed a pivot to the past memory of his father's failure to help him, linked with the idea that someone else should have helped his brother more. This pattern revealed a type of juggling ("juggling concepts about a topic" in Table 4–1) rather than effectively sequencing concepts about the topic. By switching from current to past, Mr. Beam sought to avoid a dreaded state of guilt that would be activated by associations to his brother's death because he felt that continuing with his own work despite his brother's plea for help was bad. His defensive maneuver involved a shift in time span from recent years to childhood years ("shifting time span" in Table 4–1).

We can do a partial formulation of this episode of having the image of his "bad" father. The *purpose* was to avoid arousal of his own guilty feelings and to avoid entry into a dreaded state of remorseful rumination. The *process* was to inhibit sets of ideas that evoked remorse and instead to evoke his own anger, an emotion that can reciprocally inhibit guilt. This targeting of his father rather than himself as the person to be blamed involved shifting roles ("shifting self/other roles" in Table 4–1). The *outcome* was a shift away from a potential guilty state and toward or into a state of anger because his father was the one who was behaving in a way that was uncaring and selfish.

Implications for Treatment

Recognizing important but unresolved themes and the defensive controls that are obstacles to resolving them leads to plans for treatment. For example, both Mrs. Sea and Mr. Beam were avoiding topics related to loss—Mrs. Sea's husband and Mr. Beam's brother. Heightened defensiveness when the topic was broached indicated the unresolved problems. As therapists, we could plan to counteract this inhibition by directing attention to these issues dose by dose, rather than in a single overwhelming confrontation. For example, when Mrs. Sea focused excessively on near-future topics, we could ask her to consider other time frames: who she was before her loss, and who did she wish to become in the future. We could empathically join with her in recognizing why these topics were emotionally hard for her to consider and how defensiveness barred her eventual working through them. We could establish hope for systematic work to reduce discords, mismatches, and discrepancies in belief within the unresolved and conflictual themes.

As mentioned, once signs of defensive control processes are observed in relation to a specific topic, that topic is already emerging. I think it is often better to deal with partially intrusive topics than with themes that are unresolved but totally warded off, so that the patient can understand the reasons for focusing carefully and repeatedly on the theme. Exceptions to that generality occur when globally avoided topics must be faced so that the patient can make decisions. When time is important, the therapist can counteract long-term characterological avoidance patterns.

Observing the concepts and themes that a patient repeats when an emotional topic arises leads us to useful techniques of attention engagement. When a patient repeatedly touches on a theme but then cuts off elaboration of emotional concepts, we can counteract the effort to stifle expression by simply repeating the words that were cut off, followed by a pause that encourages the patient to fill in the missing end to the sentence. This technique is the bread and low-cholesterol spread of psychotherapy; we serve it up on many occasions, and there are many jokes about carrying it to ridiculous extremes. Still, it is a valuable tool when used for a purpose.

When patients juggle back and forth in concepts about a topic, while avoiding the emotionality of what lies ahead in a chain of ideas and feelings, we can ask questions that move the train of ideas forward. For example, if a patient with work anxiety symptoms has endlessly shifted back and forth between the pros and cons of planning a meeting with a boss with whom a conflictual relationship has been identified, we can say something like "Hmm, I'd like it if you would tell me exactly what you think is actually likely to happen when you meet your boss tomorrow."

This directive encourages the patient to turn attention to examining several possible scenarios: what is *actually* likely, what is *desired*, and what transactional outcomes are most *feared*. After an answer to our question, we might continue to help move a train of thought along by saying "Now that we have reviewed what is probably going to actually happen, let's contrast that with how you might imagine it turning out ideally well" and "how do you imagine this might turn out disastrously, in a way you dread even if it is quite unlikely." Having alternative scenarios clearly stated rather than avoided can lead to useful differentiations between rational and irrational thinking.

We can also counteract specific defensive control processes by interpreting them rather than counteracting them. This leaves it up to the patient whether to counteract automatic and unconscious defensive maneuvers with acts of consciously deployed intent or "will." Of course, such explicit interpretations of defensive resistances usually also carry an implicit suggestion of "doing otherwise," that is, attempting consciously to reduce the specific avoidance to which we have drawn attention. An example would be saying something like, "You are using a fantasy exploration of what might happen to avoid the painful necessity of thinking about what may really happen. That prevents you from examining realistic possibilities and exploring options for your next actions, so you will go into that meeting without a plan. If you only have fantasy ruminations, you may never evolve an effective plan that could reduce your phobia about that meeting."

Many aspects of interaction are based on implicit and procedural rather than explicit and declarative knowledge (Posner 1989; Squire 1986). The beliefs that lead to emotions and transactions are not necessarily warded off by defensive control processes, but they are not usually consciously represented. The nature of storage and activation of such knowledge makes the processes nonconscious. Representing the ideas in communication allows the use of consciousness as a special tool for altering cognitive sequences that otherwise operate automatically. In our therapeutic discourse, we can help a patient focus on, label, and reorder such concepts.

In counteracting defensive control processes, or in using conscious control processes to alter automatic functioning, we aim to help our patients recognize linkages of associated ideas, express emotions, and reorder their thinking in ways that allow them to recognize cause-and-effect sequences. We help them to examine these causations. The goal is to modify cause-and-effect reasoning and arrive at new choices of how to act.

Because the focus will be on emotionally charged topics of high importance to the patient, and because the patient will (often) have an attitude that such topics *cannot* be resolved, it is important in many cases for the therapist to counteract the patient's effort to change the topic by declaring it "over," as we saw both Mrs. Sea and Mr. Beam try to do. In addition to increasing the *hope* of resolutions and integrations, the therapist may teach patients how to keep topics open until new levels of topic completion can occur.

For example, consider a patient who has had a stressor event with an aspect of personal guilt, like Mr. Beam's sense that he had neglected his suicidal brother's plea for help. In early sessions, we will have learned to observe when he tends to leave the important theme. Before he shifts away from the topic, we can ask him a question that leads him further down a path toward resolution than he has progressed on his own. For example, we might ask "How much expiation and remorse might be required before you are forgiven for your negligence?"

In patients who defensively avoid cross-translations of meanings in different modes of communication, we can counteract the status quo by encouraging and emulating enrichment of meaning. If our patient gives only nonverbal, bodily signals and paralinguistic communication of certain emotions and interpersonal gambits, we can model how to use explicit words for such communications. We speak the previously unspeakable. Part of our modeling shows that expression on difficult topics can occur in a well-modulated state of mind, rather than a hyperexcited, undermodulated, or rigidly restrained state. We show that clear speech is not followed now by scorn, rejection, or criticism, which the patient may have experienced from others in the past. The patient can learn how to speak the hitherto unspeakable and gain a useful level of control over what previously was automatically avoided.

Character Defenses

As we plan treatment for a patient with a personality disorder, inference of habitual defensive styles is often a valuable aspect of formulation. These defensive styles may function in ways that have warded off some insults and helped the patient achieve control over passions and external dangers, but kept the patient from learning from life experiences (Horowitz 1992; Shapiro 1965). That is why Reich (1949) called habitual defenses "character armor." Change may require knowing why learning from life experiences has not occurred. Techniques to gradually counteract maladaptive character defenses may be used to allow the patient to learn from new experiences.

The goal in long-term therapy may be to foster more mature character development. In shorter-term crisis-oriented treatments, the goal may be to counteract habitual defensive avoidances enough to work through acute problems and restore a pre-crisis equilibrium. For this purpose, certain styles may be related to specific techniques.

As I have discussed in more detail elsewhere (Horowitz 1991, 1993, 1995a, 1997), the global and impressionistic style of histrionic patients can be countered by efforts to get at details, the unemotional generalizations of the compulsive style can be countered by pointing attention to the emotional heart of a topic instead of to peripheral details, and the sliding of values by a narcissistic patient scan be coun-tered by tactful deflations of self-aggrandizing distortions. Some of these approaches to obstacles in therapy to relieve crises are summa-rized in Table 4–3, Table 4–4, and Table 4–5.

Recognizing conflictual themes and repetitive signs of defensive control processes leads to the formulation of where to focus and what potential obstacles to expect. We begin with a question: How and why do avoidances and distortions of certain topics occur? Then we may ask ourselves: Is the present defensive state caused by intense stress, or do the signs we observe indicate habitual limitations on rational information processing? If the barriers are habitual, we can ask: Where did the styles of defense come from? Why has the patient not learned more adaptive forms of understanding and planning?

In either event, we engage in answering these questions: What emotional dangers are warded off? Are there internal as well as ex-ternal sources of threat, unconscious as well as conscious ones? The next step of formulation helps us answer these questions by giving us specific configurations of beliefs as they concern conflicts and deficits in identity, relationships, and character.

Table 4–3.   Some obstacles to clarity in histrionic personality disorders and their counteractants in therapy

Defensive style	Therapeutic counter
Global or selective inattention with impressionistic rather than accurate discourse	Encourage talk and provide verbal labels; ask for details, then construct cause-and-effect sequences in stories.
Limiting disclosure by inhibition of ideas	Encourage verbal production through frequent repetitions and clarifications.
Short circuit to rapid but often erroneous conclusions	Keep subject open; refocus attention in a context of support.
Misinterpretations based on person-schematic stereo-types, deflecting from appraisal of reality to assumptions about wishes and fears	Interpret what is likely and contrast that with what is dreaded and desired; differentiate reality from fantasy and current time frames from past time frames.

Table 4–4. Some obstacles to clarity in compulsive personality disorders and their counteractants in therapy

Defensive style	Therapeutic counter
Excessively detailed but peripheral discourse	Ask for central impressions, relevance to self, and emotional reactions.
Avoiding disclosure of emotions; exceptionally "verbal"	Interpret linkage of emotional meanings to ideational meanings; focus attention on specific memories, fantasies, and felt bodily sensations.
Juggling opposing sets of meanings on a topic, back and forth	Hold to one valence of a topic; interpret reasons for defensive juggling.
Endless rumination without reaching decisions	Encourage imagination of reaching decisions and ideas about what a specific possible decision then implies.

Table 4–5. Some obstacles to clarity in narcissistic personality disorders and their counteractants in therapy

Defensive style	Therapeutic counter
Excessive focus of attention on praise and blame	Avoid being provoked into either praising or blaming, yet realistically bolster self-esteem.
Denial of "wounding" information	Use tactful timing and wording to counteract denials; identify and challenge irrational beliefs about inferiority or need for perfection to feel worthwhile.
Sliding meanings	Consistently define meanings and encourage realistic attributions of blame.
Overbalance in finding routes to self-enhancement	While bolstering a sense of competence by emphasizing skills, cautiously deflate grandiosities.
Dislocated attributes of the self or another person	Clarify who is who in terms of intentions.
Quick forgiveness of self	Point out corruptions (tactfully); model how to act as a noncorrupt person with responsible commitments.

Chapter 5

IDENTITY, RELATIONSHIPS, AND DYSFUNCTIONAL BELIEFS

This step of formulation is especially important for patients who repeat maladaptive interpersonal patterns. The goal is to understand and modify their dysfunctional beliefs about identity and relationships. Although patients may consciously know some irrational attitudes, they may not be conscious of how they link beliefs together in forming intentions and expectations. They may not realize that when planning how to attain personal goals, they base decisions on illusions.

By differentiating realistic beliefs from fantasy-based beliefs, we can help a patient develop a sense of coherent and competent identity even in the midst of stressful life circumstances. We can help a patient reduce repetitions. The first three steps of formulation have already designated certain patterns; now our task is to ask: Why do dysfunctional repetitions occur? What would be useful for a patient to learn to change?

These questions are typically difficult for patients to answer independently. In conjunction with a therapist, however, a patient may be able to make sense of why dysfunctional but repeated patterns have occurred. Determining why repetitions occur and what changes can be made requires clarifying facts and then establishing casual connections between the facts.

Cause-and-effect sequences are the kind of connections between facts that patients frequently obscure. They do not consciously see how certain events and expressions lead to other events and expressions. They may consciously know what happened but not why and how. We can clarify the why and how linkages.

This process of clarification of connections is helped by use of a conceptual tool. The tool is a model of how self and other are connected by roles and transactional sequences. This tool is called a role relationship model, and it embodies cause-and-effect beliefs. Any individual has many role relationship models as part of memory-stored personal meaning systems. Each role relationship model carries meanings about who is involved and what they mean to do (Horowitz 1979/1987, 1989, 1991).

Constructing role relationship models puts together a combination of beliefs. This construction requires both pattern recognition and clinical inference. We check and revise our inferences. They can be wrong or off the mark. Each role relationship model helps us observe more clearly, and as we observe more, we change our model to better fit patterned repetitions.

A set, or configuration, of role relationship models can clarify a patient's complex and even contradictory ideas about self and others. A patient seeking treatment seldom has just one, or just a few, erroneous beliefs. Models and configurations allow us to see connections and antitheses between these beliefs. By using them, we are able to define more clearly the ambivalence, conundrums, dilemmas, conflicts, and discords of value that may lie at the root of problems.

We clarified complex state shifts and cycles in the second step of formulation and clarified further by considering some states as ways to ward off defensively other more dreaded states. Now, we go further by explaining what configurations of beliefs led the patient to enter each state. The core beliefs we aim to infer are about roles, expectations, and intentions. These beliefs may be explicit or implicit, declarative or procedural. They function as conscious and unconscious assumptions about how people deal with each other.

Once we have inferred repetitive beliefs, we can select and counteract core distortions. These are the irrational attitudes that lead to dysfunctional interpersonal behaviors and distressing lapses in self-esteem. We use clarifications, interpretations, and suggestions to modify recurrent errors. We help the patient to be more adaptive, rational, and objective about identity; more resilient in planning actions; and more sagacious in making assumptions about the intentions of others.

When needed, we provide support by giving information about how the world may actually work. We also support the self-esteem of patients as they experiment with new ways of asserting themselves with others.

As just mentioned, our approach involves explaining states of mind by defining role relationship models for each state already described. Clinical research has shown that such formulations can be done reliably and with predictive validity using the system presented here. Clinicians independently reviewing recordings of sessions can reach a consensus on their inferences using role relationship models as a format for putting together beliefs (Eells et al. 1995; Horowitz and Eells 1993; Horowitz et al. 1995b). In this chapter, I show you how to construct such role relationship models.

Link to the Previous Steps of Formulation

Your way is partially paved by the pieces collected during the earlier steps of the formulation process. Pieces from the first step include a listing of symptoms, such as identity disturbances, depersonalization, or social problems (e.g., lack of assertiveness). From the second step, you have information about how each state contains special views about self and others, such as an irrationally weak view of self during unassertive states. From the third step, you have relevant topics of concern and styles of warding off certain emotional memories or fantasies. Instead of thinking through a topic of worry about lack of work success, the patient may always say "I don't know what to do" to avoid thinking of the emotional consequences of each alternative route of action.

For example, problematic *phenomena* for a patient may have included excessive social assertions of grandeur. *States of mind* may have included cycles ranging from chaotic depersonalization to a state characterized by belief in personal omnipotence, with a related irrational appraisal of others as stupid and pathetic. A state where others were viewed as envious, powerful, and intending to persecute the self may have been part of the cycle. The *topics of concern* may have included work mistakes and questions of whether to plan revenge on others. *Obstacles to clarity* may have been noted, such as shifting blame for mistakes away from the self onto others. Now, irrational beliefs about cause and effect will be identified, including connections between beliefs in inferiority, superiority, and the reason for and consequences of work mistakes. Role relationship models involved in grandiosity would be linked to motives to avoid self-deflation and the dreaded state of chaos in a sense of identity.

Listening

As you listen to what a patient reports, and observe how he or she reacts, you note behaviors that indicate maladaptive beliefs. Your mind, with training, will begin to summarize the core irrational elements automatically. Eventually in treatment, you will help the patient to compare and contrast these with more rational alternatives.

Your first step is a low-level clinical inference. What the patient says or does is repeated in your own mind with only one addition. Usually, the addition is a connection between concepts. Usually, that connection has to do with a similarity—teacher is like father—or with a cause-and-effect sequence—only if I am always grateful and never angry will my teacher help me. Key words in linking beliefs are *if, then, but, because,* and *so.* For instance: *If* I am always grateful, *then* my teacher will help me, *but* if I am ever angry, *then* my teacher will leave me *because* my father did, and teacher is like father, *so* I must stifle any hostile responses.

Inference

We are now at a period of psychotherapy integration. Previously diverse schools of practice now converge in theory about how to form low-level clinical inferences. All schools agree that irrational or dysfunctional beliefs exist within mental structure, and that in some persons these contribute to symptom formation and personality problems. Psychodynamic (Horowitz 1979/1987), control-mastery (Silberschatz et al. 1991), cognitive (Persons 1992), and behavioral (Goldfried 1996) theorists agree on a good way to infer and summarize core problematic beliefs. This agreed-on framework uses the if, then, but, because, and so sequence.

For example, here is a way you might state an observed repetition of a dysfunctional belief: "*If* I pursue success in my own in my career, *then* my mother will abandon me *because* she feels betrayed if I go beyond her level achievement; *but if* I remain less successful than she, *then* she will stay warmly close to me, *so* I will procrastinate to avoid being too successful." Such a belief may lead to anxiety, personal inhibition, or guilt. It could, in part, explain why a career success led to symptom formation rather than joy. The warded-off emotions within a topic of concern, such as procrastination at work, could include guilt (hurting mother), fear and despair (losing mother), and shame (failing at work). By clarifying the beliefs, the surprising negative emotion (guilt, fear) on success might be understood. Then, the dilemma behind the procrastination can be confronted, challenged, and modified.

Configurations of Beliefs

Summaries of core beliefs can help you construct larger and more explanatory models. A patient will often link contradictory beliefs in a network of meanings about self and others. I call these arrangements configurations of role relationship models to emphasize the connected assembly of associational linkages. These links may include those between seemingly antithetical or polar-opposite beliefs. The whole is an entanglement that has been hard for the patient to unravel.

Role relationship models are mental schematizations of persons that include emotions and scripts for transaction. The ingredients in such models include

1. role of *self*
2. role of *others*
3. intention and *action,* including expression of emotion

    a. that can *initiate* a transactional sequence
    b. that occur in *response* and *reaction*
    c. that occur as actions *actually expressed* or those only *thought* or fantasied

4. *critical evaluation* of action and intention

You will find ingredients in three domains: stories about current problems (at work, in caretaking, in intimate relationships, or in other social activities); contents of important, recurring memories and fantasies about the past with significant others; and with you (how the patient presents and provokes in the domain of social alliances, therapeutic alliances, and relationships of transference and countertransference).

For instance, a graduate student who misinterpreted the emotional proclivities of a mentor may be repeating a past pattern and may be likely to repeat it again in the treatment. As such a patient discusses producing work for a mentor, he or she might report a recurrent state cycle that had, as its worst component, a dreaded state of *frantic anguish*. Each episode of frantic anguish may have been precipitated when expecting to meet with the mentor. Several stories about such anticipations may help establish a pattern. In each story, the graduate student would occupy a role of *needy and inferior supplicate* to a *superior professor regarded as selfish and manipulative*. When the student sought guidance and help, the mentor might use the need to exploit the student. A hostile reaction to the expected exploitation might tend to occur, but the student also expected anger at being exploited to lead to *abandonment* by a figure essential in conferring a degree. The dreaded consequence would be personal demoralization, self-disgust, shame, and helpless pining for necessary but unavailable help. These repeated beliefs can be condensed into a role relationship model for the state of frantic anguish, as shown at the bottom of Figure 5–1.

Other stories might show other roles and transactional sequences with the mentor. By abstracting out patterns, you will soon have several role relationship models. These may be assembled into a configuration by considering which role relationship models are desired, dreaded, or serve as compromises for wish-fear or approach-avoidance dilemmas. Using a familiar format, as shown in Figure 5–2, allows you to put alternative role relationship models together into a configuration. Various self-concepts are now shown within a central circle of self-organization.

A role relationship model configuration is a model of motivation and meanings about self as related to other(s). The desired role relationship model in the lower-right quadrant can be linked in a network

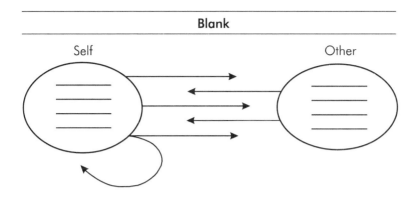

Blank

Self   Other

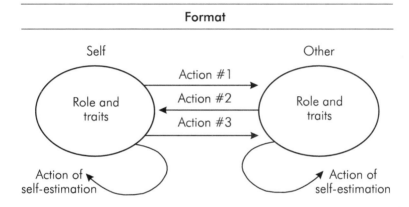

Format

Self   Other

Role and   Role and
traits   traits

Action #1
Action #2
Action #3

Action of   Action of
self-estimation   self-estimation

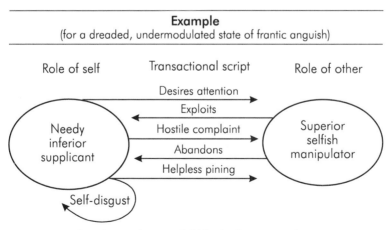

Example
(for a dreaded, undermodulated state of frantic anguish)

Role of self   Transactional script   Role of other

Needy   Desires attention   Superior
inferior   Exploits   selfish
supplicant   Hostile complaint   manipulator
                      Abandons
                      Helpless pining

Self-disgust

Figure 5–1. Role relationship model blank, format, and an example.

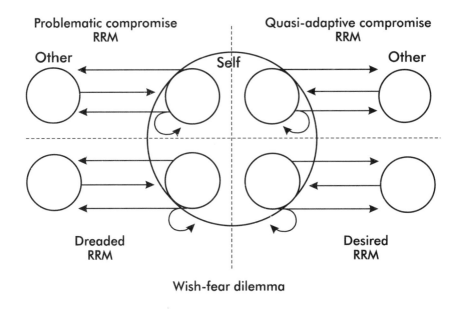

Figure 5–2.   Blank configuration of role relationship models (RRMs).

of associations to feared consequences in the dreaded role relationship model of the lower-left quadrant. The lower half of a role relationship model configuration may contain a repeated dilemma, a crucial connection that causes an unresolvable conflict. The top half contains compromise role relationship models activated to ward off the dilemma, and the danger of entry into the dreaded state.

Problematic states were identified during the second step of the formulation process. These states may stem from observations made during the first step because these states frequently contain the first complaints of our patients. For that reason, problematic states are in the upper-left quadrant, the "first-to-be-read" part of a configuration of a role relationship model.

Quasi-adaptive compromises, represented in the upper-right quadrant, have less negative affect. Although quasi-adaptive because they are associated with states of lessened distress, these role relationship models are a defensive compromise because they do not reach a satisfying goal. A general role relationship model configuration illustrates these role relationship model placements; see Figure 5–3.

For a further example of how to infer role relationship models, we return to the case of Mrs. Sea.

As you may recall, I summarized several states of mind for Mrs. Sea in Table 3–3. That configuration of states had a desired state *(happily excited)*, a dreaded state *(agony of grief)*, a problematic compromise *(struggle with grief)*, and a quasi-adaptive compromise *(cool and poised)*. Now, we can add self-concepts that occur more frequently in each of these states. These views of self are determined by noting the types of words Mrs. Sea uses to describe herself. In her *agony of grief,* she dreaded self-concepts as a bereft, emotionally uncontrolled woman. As we will see from further material, she viewed herself as unreliable and selfish as well as bereft. She tried to stifle the agony in her *struggle with grief,* but still felt vulnerable. She was tempted to avoid relationships in which she might be vulnerable by stabilizing herself as a career woman, concentrating on developing her independence, and maintaining a stoic demeanor. In this way, she tried to maintain her *cool and poised* state. This did not satisfy her wish to be a vibrant woman, capable of happiness and excitement. This configu-

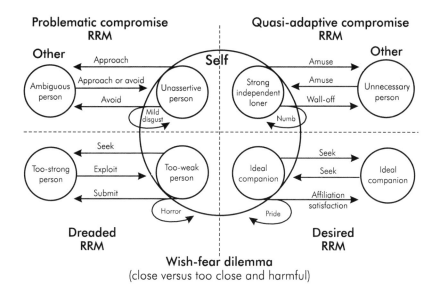

Figure 5–3.   Configuration of role relationship models (RRMs): a general example.

ration of different possible identities as related to some of her states of mind is shown in Figure 5–4.

These views were part of an important theme, yearning for the kind of intimacy she had shared with James, her now dead husband. Mrs. Sea had an opportunity to renew that kind of relationship with Sydney. She was involved with him in a new dating experience, and he seemed safe and attractive. Yet, in some states, intimacy with Sidney became dangerous rather than exciting because she still unconsciously schematized James as alive. She viewed her feelings with Sidney as if she were cheating on James. Automatically regarding her new intimacy as infidelity led to potential emotions of fear, guilt, shame, and doubt. Defensive avoidance of this conflictual theme prevented entry into dreaded states.

After a number of sessions, her avoidance maneuvers were reduced. It was possible to infer her self-concepts around the topic of concern of this new intimate relationship. A configuration of a role relationship model for this topic of concern is provided in Figure 5–5.

At first, it will seem artificial and complicated to construct role relationship models and configurations for your patients. If you try, however, you may soon find you can listen more carefully to discourse as it relates to identity and relationship issues. What happens is this:

Problematic "struggle with grief" state	Quasi-adaptive "cool and poised" state
• Vulnerable woman	• Stoic independent woman
• Bereft, emotionally uncontrolled, unreliable, and selfish woman	• Vibrant woman
Dreaded "agony of grief" state	Desired "happily excited" state

Figure 5–4. Configuration of self-concepts of Mrs. Sea.

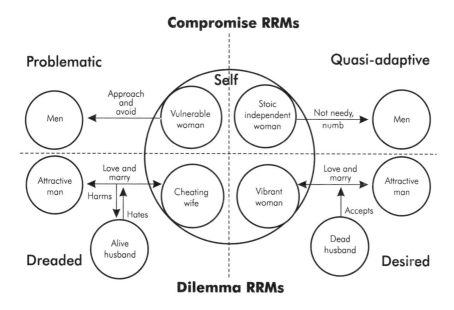

Figure 5–5. Role relationship model (RRM) configuration for Mrs. Sea.

you learn to listen for a sequence of transactions, and you note when shifts in roles occur. That helps you understand shifts in states and repetitions in state cycles.

It will help to show you a concrete example of how to construct a role relationship model from a segment of a clinical session. We take a patient's speech and place it into a format that helps us infer a role relationship model. We use a format that starts with the self and goes back and forth, in a sequence of interactions with another person. The roles of self and other are given in terms of characteristics or attributes that explain the style and content of the transaction. This format can be stated as a map for a sentence:

"I, who am like this, did thus to a person, who is like this, and that person responded by doing thus and I then felt like this."

Mrs. Sea said this about her new intimate relationship:

I went for a weekend with Sidney, and it started out to be happy and exciting for me. Just when I wanted to enjoy how good I looked for the first time in a long time and what a fine man he really is, I suddenly thought of James. I felt, I don't know why, it seems so irrational. I felt very, very badly. Like I was a cheater.

A paraphrase according to our map comes out like this:

> I, who am a good-looking woman, was happy and excited with Sidney, who is a fine man, and then I felt like a cheater who felt bad about James.

Having observed the pattern, one might infer that she views James as accusing her of cheating. Indeed, she says this later on. Then, the paraphrase can be altered a bit into the form of if, then, and because that we discussed as a way of summarizing core beliefs:

> If I, a good-looking woman, want to feel happy and excited with Sidney, a fine man, then I will remember I am wife to James and feel badly about cheating, because I value fidelity [to James].

As a result of the self loving Sidney, she imagines hurting James and she enters a guilty state of mind.

The roles of Sidney and James in this dilemma are reversible. She can also feel guilty about Sidney when she retains her identity as intimate only with James. You will observe this attitude in the following discourse.

> For some reason I was thinking yesterday about what, how I would feel, I mean, if I could bring him [James] back, if I could go back and somehow turn back the clock and just go back 2 years [before the death] and start over. But in order to do that would mean of course erasing Sidney, and I mean honestly, I felt, yeah, I would still go back. I would still rather have that life than this life, and that, that didn't make me very happy either. I mean a little part of me felt relieved that I felt that way, but then I thought that's not very fair to Sidney. . . . But I still feel a little guilty that I, that I would go back if I could. . . . And maybe it's just that there's more time invested in that than what I have now. I don't know that I honestly loved James anymore than I love Sidney. I love Sidney a great deal. But you know James was, I don't know, James was a life, you know, James was everything to me. And I don't know Sidney and I are new enough, I guess that I could. That I would go back if I could. But in a way I guess I'm glad that it's a choice I don't have to make. It would be incredibly difficult to hurt Sidney.

A paraphrase is:

> If I, James's wife, remain as if still married to James and give up
> Sidney, who would be hurt, then I would feel guilty toward Sidney
> because I value fidelity [to Sidney].

She wanted to feel good, attractive, and loving. She could be in
a *happily excited* state were she to stabilize this self-concept as a free,
vibrant, sexual, and responsible woman. But she could not stabilize
this state. She tended to lose her excitement and pride, which resulted
in a state transition into *agony of grief* when with Sidney. She had
intrusive ideas that she was cheating on James, her dead husband. She
missed him terribly. She might then try to ward off the agony and
cycle into her *struggle with grief* state. She would worry that she had
been too dependent on James and was now pining too much for a
husband. She would also worry that she might become dependent on
Sidney, the new man, were they to remain intimate and eventually marry.

These concepts made her feel tense rather than agonized. Although distressing and problematic, a ruminative state of struggling
with alternative aims was preferable to the undermodulated state of
agony of grief. But she could feel more comfortable by entering into
a *cool and poised* state, as organized by her unloving but stoically
independent self-concept. Yet this was lonely; her desires were not
met. Her cycle of states tended to repeat a search for happiness and
assertion of herself as a vibrant woman. A configuration of role relationship models for this cycle on the topic of intimacy shows the key
conflicts (see Figure 5–5).

Intimacy and possible marriage with Sidney conflicted with Mrs.
Sea's idea of being the loyal and loving wife of a living James. If she
loved Sidney, she felt she was cheating James. This formulation allows
us to anticipate a possible route of change in treatment. Although she
consciously knew James was dead, she unconsciously generated
moods on the basis of her unconscious schematizations of James as if
yet alive. Her identity concepts were still linked strongly to her many
associational linkages that still declared her attachment to James. With
more work in mourning, she could conceptualize James as really, and
safely, dead. Then she could imagine herself as the loving wife of
Sidney without fear that she was cheating on James.

Even if she imagined James watching her from heaven, she could still come to view him as approving a restoration of her own life as a woman. Once she had reschematized James as safely dead, she could remember the love and marriage between herself and James without experiencing James as a rival of Sidney or herself as trespassing against her important value of fidelity. This potential change in her enduring and slowly changing structure of deep beliefs is shown in Figure 5–6.

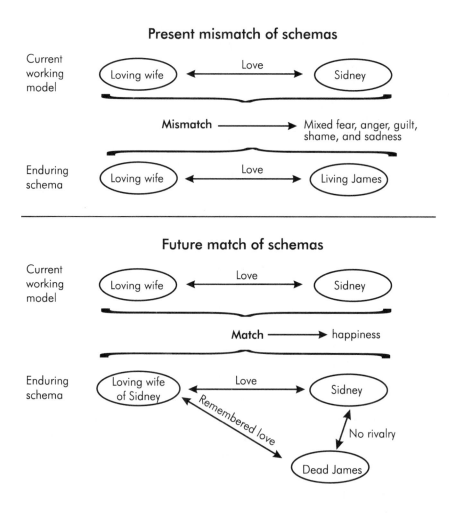

Figure 5–6.   Present conflict and future resolution of conflict for Mrs. Sea.

Steps of Formulation for Mrs. Sea

We can now consider an overall treatment plan for the psychotherapy of Mrs. Sea. I will repeat some items from earlier steps of formulation.

☐ Phenomena

- Label and explain her intrusive and avoidant experiences as phases in her mourning process, one that is not yet completed.
- Emphasize realistic hope for restoration of her sense of happiness after she works through grief to completion.

☐ States

- When she seems about to shift into undermodulated states, slow down her ideation by repetitions and organizing combinations in such a way as to avoid emotional flooding.
- Provide her with empathic support during shimmering states.
- Stabilize her working states by modeling dose-by-dose discourse on emotional topics.
- Focus her attention to reduce her shifts into overmodulated states.

☐ Topics of Concern and Defensive Control
   Processes

- Counteract her avoidance maneuver of disavowal, switching topics, and short-circuiting to premature closures (by shifting time frames).
- Identify her unresolved grief as a focal topic of concern and link this to other such topics: her future identity and her new intimacy.
- Label her nonverbal emotional signs and state how and why she stifles verbal statements of emotion.
- Interpret the importance of her warded-off ideas and show how her conflicts can be safely contemplated during the treatment sessions.

☐ Identity, Role Relationship Models, and Dysfunctional Beliefs

- Interpret how and why her enduring, unconscious, but procedurally active schema of James as alive conflicts with her developing her new intimacy.
- Use and repeat metaphor of James as "safely dead."
- Help her to integrate her discrepant views of self as vibrant woman and as cheater.

More complex examples of how to use role relationship models in formulating disorders of personality are given elsewhere (Horowitz 1991, 1992, 1994). I do wish to comment briefly, however, on the theoretical background to this approach.

Person Schemas Theory

The system for inferring role relationship models is based on person schemas theory. This theory acknowledges that each person may have multiple self-concepts as aspects of unconscious procedural knowledge. This, in turn, can lead to a sense of varying conscious identity. The sense of "I," of other, and of "me in a relationship" changes, sometimes in cyclic maladaptive patterns. In these patterns, there are varied views of what intentions, expectations, and transactional sequences will be enacted. Because variations from state to state may be anticipated in unconscious conditioned associations and information processing, a person's unconscious repertoire of self and other schemas may be defensively controlled.

The anticipation of dreaded states of mind, such as identity chaos, harmful impulsive action, abject terror, utter despair, or intolerable shame and guilt, may be an aspect of unconscious information processing. The effect of defensive facilitations and inhibitions of various organized belief structures about self and other can lead to the activation of meanings that organize alternative, compromise states. Some of these states manifest symptoms and problems, but despite this distress, the states are held in place to avoid entry into even more dreaded states or even more dangerously impulsive acting out of harmful actions.

The automatic repetition of maladaptive forms of conditioned associations may be altered by use of consciousness as a special tool for choices that lead to change. Focused attention, declarative transformations of key beliefs, and determined practices of new behaviors can lead to new conditioned associations, new procedural knowledge, and an eventual alteration of habitual automatic processing. This complex task of change may involve insight, new subjective understanding of evoked feelings in conscious information processing, and new decisions that affect current and future emotional relationships.

Such theory is described more fully elsewhere (Horowitz 1979/1987, 1988a, 1988b, 1991a, in press; Horowitz et al. 1996). It is rooted in concepts of transference (S. Freud 1912a), personal constructs (Kelly 1955), object relations (Kernberg 1968; Winnicott 1953), attachment theory (Bowlby 1969, 1988), self psychology (Kohut 1977; Markus 1977), and learning theory (for behavioral automatisms) (Lazarus 1991). Lewin (1935) emphasized respective roles of self and other, Berne (1961, 1964, 1972) used that format for inferring self-other beliefs in various "ego-states," and Murray (1938) and Erikson (1954) analyzed configurations of possible self-identities with thematic polarities. All viewed self and other representations as usually unconscious memory residues of prior experiences, including ones based on childhood attachments and ones based on fantasy connected with reality (Bowlby 1988).

Person schemas have also been called transference templates (S. Freud 1912a), plans (Miller et al. 1960), scripts (Berne 1961, 1964, 1972), nuclear scenes (Tomkins 1978), core conflictual relationship themes (Luborsky and Crits-Christoph 1990), cognitions (A. T. Beck 1976), cognitive schemas (Kovacs and Beck 1978; Lichtenberg 1975; Slap and Saykin 1983), and unconscious fantasies (Arlow 1969). Singer and Salovey (1991) provide a review. A connectionist view provides a substrate-neutral basis for person schemas as a set of linkages between information (Rumelhart and McClelland 1986); associational strengths may be flexibly altered during parallel distributive processing (Stinson and Palmer 1991).

Person schemas theory led to the formalization of procedures for inferring role relationship models and configurations (Horowitz 1989, 1991). The system presented here was found reliable in empirical studies (Eells et al. 1995; Horowitz and Eells 1993; Horowitz et al. 1995). In one study, early role relationship model configurations predicted later transference dilemmas (Horowitz et al. 1995b).

The advantage of summarizing patterns into several role relationship models is that, as a result, we have a set of repetitive self-identities for our patients, each as embedded in relationship views. Our patients have a finite set of such identities and relationship models. This set is a repertoire of their potential beliefs. Some are more irrational and dysfunctional than others. We can define them and seek to help patients to modify these "pathogenic" aspects of their repertoire and the motivations that activate these elements. We also seek to help patients associate disparate components into new, supraordinate schemas of self and other.

In helping patients to develop new and integrated belief structures, including a realistically competent sense of identity and effectiveness, we need to realize that we are dealing with both conscious and nonconscious sources of personal knowledge, relationship attachments, social skills, and emotionality. All of these are influenced by the contents and integrations of this personal knowledge. It also helps us to understand that person schemas are used by the mind to fill in missing items of interpersonal information.

Person schemas quicken responses but carry a liability. They produce errors in understanding others, and they can result in patterned, repeated mistakes in action. These errors and mistakes occur as our patient constructs inner working models of social situations. These working models combine perceptions of current situations and beliefs from activated role relationship models. This dynamic construction of operating knowledge is illustrated in Figure 5–7.

This figure illustrates how an actual social transaction shapes, and is shaped by, inner intentions and expectations (Horowitz 1988a). The dominance of one of several potential role relationship models from a personal repertoire is shown by the *bold arrow*. The other enduring schemas might produce alternative states of mind, but they have less influence in the current state. Nonetheless, in unconscious processing—or consciously, during shimmering states—other role relationship models may affect thinking and feeling. This happens in the course of nonconscious parallel processing. If an alternative schema achieved a better fit to perceptions and approvals, it might become the dominant role relationship model. This shift to a different

Social transactions

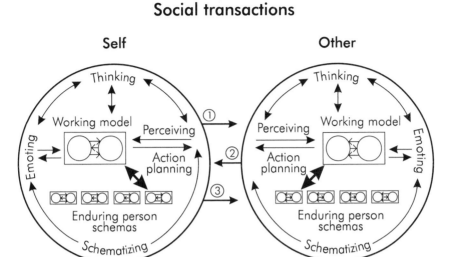

Figure 5–7. Social situations are shaped by activation of person schemas and vice versa.

role relationship model could alter state and lead to cyclic repetitions. Intentions, expectations, mood, behavioral expressions, and the state of the other person might all shift as a consequence of the shift in active person schematization, or role relationship model.

For example, a patient may be in a state of feeling worthwhile and safe, experiencing self as competent and the therapist as interested, expert, and understanding. This patient may, however, be exquisitely sensitive to slights. Noting a slight shift in the gaze of the therapist, to a clock for example, the patient may unconsciously shift activity of enduring role relationship models and his or her current working model. Now the patient feels incompetent and unworthy and views the therapist as only feigning interest. This dreaded role relationship model produces distress, and it may be warded off by yet another shift. Now, the patient reverses roles and activates a role relationship model of self as dismissive of and disinterested in the therapist, who is now viewed as incompetent and unworthy. This negativity might have been dormant, inhibited earlier in the hour when the patient felt worthwhile and safe.

Psychotherapy Technique

This step of formulation helps us clarify conflicts, irrationalities, and maladaptive behavioral patterns. We can use it to help patients focus on contradictory attitudes or self-impairing actions, to revise beliefs and actions, and to plan and practice new styles of expression and action.

The patient operating alone, before the therapy, will have been stymied by hopelessness, misunderstanding, or defensive avoidance of the emotional response to fixed personal dilemmas. The safety and know-how operating within a therapeutic alliance allows new or renewed processing of social information, but the patient usually discovers this only gradually. The discovery itself develops new person schemas.

A patient examines the interpretations of the therapist and interprets the therapist's intention and expectation. Increased conscious awareness of how a working model influences his or her actions begins to occur. The therapist may hear the patient say "I didn't realize I was so resentful of you until you pointed it out." This increased awareness can be carried over to other relationships.

Contradictory attitudes usually require tactful and repeated confrontation. The careful statement of two or more beliefs is required. One asks the patient to compare this with that. Challenges to compare this with that clarify *both* the more maladaptive roles *and* potential, more adaptive, roles of self. Immature, distorted views are contrasted with mature, undistorted appraisals. Through gradual changes, the patient's internal working models increasingly begin to resemble actual social situations or objective opportunities.

As the patient develops conceptual skills that assess beliefs and feelings clearly, he or she can think new ideas and feel clearer emotions. He or she can replace transference-based feelings with more appropriate ones and better regulate impulses. Conscious thought and verbal communication improve. Previously unthinkable topics can be examined to differentiate reality and fantasy. A step-by-step sequence toward satisfying goals may be learned. More fulfillment can powerfully counteract negative mood states such as depression.

Patients who are less well organized find it very difficult to progress in a step-by-step sequence. In addition, they may develop, or even come with, unrealistic transference intentions or expectations. Even during the seemingly safe situation of expert psychotherapy, they are vulnerable to states of mind dominated by elements embedded in immature and even bizarre role relationship models. Both self-control and a therapeutic alliance are difficult to maintain. When the therapist offers a possible "more objective view," the patient may feel stung, as if by criticism. The therapist is trying to point out problems, give suggestions, and interpret cause-and-effect sequences, but the patient feels badly. Some patients have a relevant cognitive deficit; they seem less able than others to update their mental models of self and others. They have a poor tolerance of ambivalence and contradiction in social circumstances. Any slight or lapse in empathy is generalized to mean intent to abandon. Even good empathy can be regarded as the dawn of a new love or hate relationship.

Such disturbances are found in some patients with borderline personality disorders. They may have a deficit in ability to connect complex meaning structures into supraordinate concepts of identity and relatedness. Instead, they tend to dissociate, split, and segregate role relationship models into all-good and all-bad configurations. For this reason, formulation may also usefully include assessment of a patient's ability to have complex views, views that can contain contradictions. If patients interpret events in a simplistic and potentially fragmenting manner, very slow and tactful actions may replace bolder therapeutic acts of interpretation. In such cases, a slow, patient, and repetitive approach may be essential to support the patient's more adaptive states. The vital issue concerns focus of attention and depth of focus of attention. Deciding on the most helpful level of focus for each patient, and for each phase of work with that patient, is the major topic in the next chapter.

Summary

Role relationship models include roles of self and others, and add scripts that are intended and expected sequences of social interaction. Desired, dreaded, or defensive compromise states may have different role relationship models. Even very complex dilemmas of relationship can be gradually clarified and confronted by using configurations of such models.

Chapter 6

PLANNING PSYCHOTHERAPY ON THE BASIS OF FORMULATIONS

We have covered four steps of formulation and considered some aspects of how each step links to technique. In this final step of formulation, we form an overall treatment plan. We consider what causes symptoms and problems. We ask: What can change? This includes change in biological, social, and psychological factors. We then act with a coordination of efforts.

At the level of phenomena, we consider the value of naming and explaining symptoms to patients. In some cases, it will be important to do this with members of a social group to reduce stigmatization and increase understanding and acceptance. At the level of states, we consider the value of techniques to reduce undercontrolled states and prevent dangerous state cycles. In some cases, we do this with medication, in others with a safe social milieu, in others with early psychotherapy interventions, and in others with a combined biopsychosocial approach.

Above All, Do No Harm

The steps of formulation involving defensiveness and deep-seated but irrational beliefs about the self and others present unique dilemmas when integrating possible techniques into a treatment plan. Some patients need their defenses even when they operate as obstacles to clarity. Undefensive conscious recognition would be emotionally overwhelming. Other patients do well with a rapid approach to revelation of usually warded-off aspects of topics of concern, provided that it is done in a safe therapeutic alliance. Following the rule "above all, do no harm" means careful consideration of how deep to go and how fast with each patient. In this chapter, I aim to provide you with some tools for conceptualizing the answers to these questions.

Capacity for Coherence in Sense of Self Over Time

People maintain varying levels of understanding of self-organization, which leads to a sense of identity or self-regard. We have already considered how individuals may have different self-concepts in different states of mind. Some individuals learned during development how to contain this multiplicity, whereas others lack this capacity and have less coherence of self (Horowitz 1995b).

Without coherence of self-organization, a person is more likely to form symptoms, have explosive shifts in state, express unstable state cycles, and experience more distortions in interpreting acts of self and other. Such people may seem to have inappropriate divisions in personal meanings, such as all-good or all-bad clusters. For this reason, low-coherence in self-organization has been called "narcissistic vulnerability" (Kernberg 1968).

As we gain experience with patients in treatment, we become better able to infer their levels of personal development. This inference goes beyond a current assessment of problems, knowledge, and skills to include estimates of the degree of co-organization, integration, or containment of various aspects of personal meanings and motives.

Self-coherence is not just a matter of motives and interpersonal style. It includes abilities to be consistent over time, as well as virtues such as personality and integrity. Consider, as an example, a person who wants attention and uses theatrical emotional displays to get it in interpersonal settings. This motive and style can be entirely normal if used with integrity. It can be neurotic if it is conflicted and either self-impairing or too manipulative of others. A person who has a loss of coherence in sense of identity might use this style to regain equilibrium by getting others to minister to the self. A person frantic with a sense of falling apart, after a perceived abandonment, may desperately demand attention in a way that destroys support systems (Horowitz 1991). Different persons displaying "histrionic emotionality" might require a very different set of therapeutic techniques.

People with low self-coherence tend to misinterpret relationships that might otherwise be helpful. They may have explosive shifts into hostile states. In contrast, people with high self-coherence are softer and less off-putting. They get irritable with frustration, but not enraged and irrationally blaming. They can soften ambivalence to others by remembering the good with the bad and can tolerate news about the self that is unpleasant.

The psychologically rich tend to get richer. People with higher levels of self-coherence over time are able to use brief treatment. They are more grateful for help and use helping facilities more adeptly. They are better able to use interpretations and challenges to irrational beliefs. This has been demonstrated in empirical research: patients with a higher capacity for coherence may have better outcomes with more expressive techniques (in an expressive/supportive matrix), whereas patients with a lower capacity for coherence may have worse outcomes with more expressive techniques and better outcomes with more support (in an expressive/support matrix) (Horowitz et al. 1984b; Kernberg 1975; Piper et al. 1991; Wallerstein 1986). Formulation of a person low in self-coherence may mean planning for slower and longer treatment. Technique may involve patient repetitions of small steps and more commitment to sustaining the relationship with the patient.

The presenting picture of a patient with a poor sense of identity, many symptoms, and explosive state changes does not necessarily mean that low self-coherence is a long-standing personality trait. Stressor events challenge identity, and regressions may occur. The picture of explosive state shifts, very distorting defenses, and irrational views may be state related. That is, the person may improve rapidly as stress is reduced. For this reason, formulating levels of self-coherence is not easy: inferences may be wrong. Inferences may be revised after more experience with the patient. Some experimentation with how each patient responds to various types of intervention is usually indicated.

A General Principle

A general principle in psychotherapy technique can help us with this important problem of how fast to go, with whom, and how to avoid doing harm to patients by going too fast with patients who are vulnerable to a loss of self-cohesion. We remain at levels where the patient can tolerate emotion and work to change. We can start with presenting complaints and take an initial aim at state stabilization. When working states in therapy sessions are consistently achieved, we can deepen the focus of attention.

To meet these goals, we must first determine how to help the patient avoid impulsive actions and dreaded moods by using psychological suggestions, social supports, and/or medications. Sometimes the hope stimulated by acting to get help, and feeling understood and bolstered by initial treatment plans, may be sufficient to meet this initial goal of reducing danger from unstable states. We then work to further establish a safe relationship.

As we proceed, we continually assess our interventions: Do they work or fail to work? By helping our patients stabilize more competent self-concepts, they will usually be better able to cope with crises, conflicts, and deficits with less irrationality and less impulsiveness. Then, our technique can shift to explorations that can lead to formulations about causation of disordered functioning. Periodically, a patient may relapse into uncontrolled and dysphoric states. Our technique should then shift from explorations and efforts to secure long-term change to techniques that increase state stabilization with short-range support and, when indicated, medication and social supports.

Selection of a Focus for Attention During Psychotherapy Sessions

We ask: What topics shall we consider? When should we shift attention to other themes? This process almost always involves a gradual deepening of topics, a sequential progression from surface issues to in-depth concerns. We deal with six levels of topics in the following order:

1. Presenting complaints
2. Related social situations, biological conditions, and precipitating stressor events
3. Current dilemmas of choice between pressing alternative decisions (e.g., how to cope with precipitating crises)
4. States and repetitive state cycles associated with recurring problems
5. Conflicted themes, obstacles to treatment, and defensive control processes
6. Concerns and developmental possibilities involving identity, relationships, and character

The first phases of treatment often involve discourse with a focus of attention on current and external contexts, the first three of the six levels just listed. The middle and latter phases of treatment often progress to a focus of attention on discourse that increasingly addresses internal and developmental contexts. We review these domains; as we do so, we also consider how to interrelate time frames, how to link personal meanings associated with the current context of crisis with knowledge from the past, and beliefs about what is possible in the future.

At the top of both Table 6–1 and Table 6–2, you see these past, present, and future time frames. The first one listed is the *current situation*, that is, the patient's situation in life outside of therapy. This time span usually goes back a year or two. The next current time frame is even more immediate: it is the *therapy situation*. The therapist and patient have a chance for clear observation of ideas and feelings in the here-and-now of their discourse. The patient can immediately review short-term memory to check and reappraise his or her own views about transactions and intentions.

Next in the row is *past developmental issues*. By focusing on how problematic personal styles evolved, we can help a patient integrate his or her life story by forming personal interpretations about how current beliefs and schemas were formed. Although they may now

Table 6–1. Foci of attention in psychotherapy: external orientation

Content areas	Time focus			
	Current situation	Therapy situation	Past developmental issues	Future planning issues
Symptoms, problems, and other salient phenomena	Engage in clear description of signs, symptoms, problems, and relevant strengths.	Note when symptoms and signs occur during sessions; note when new experiences and behaviors occur.	Clarify how and why symptoms first developed.	Establish goals and prognosis for symptom change.
Recent stressful life events	Describe what precipitated problems.	Talk about expectations of treatment and how it might become stressful or stress relieving.	Explore stories of remembered early traumas and fantasies. Differentiate as possible memory from imaginative elaborations. Differentiate current meanings from past evaluations.	Plan protective and coping steps in case precipitating events recur.
Current dilemmas and choices	Examine approach and avoidance conflicts about how to respond to external pressure and situational demands.	Clarify how, when, and why the patient resists explorations of areas he or she wishes to explore, and stifles emotions he or she wants to be able to express freely.	Study the lifelong themes in the patient of habitual dilemmas and relate these, as needed, to historical, ethnic, class, gender, or familial themes.	Make specific plans for choosing between various alternative futures.

Table 6–2. Foci of attention in psychotherapy: internal orientation

| Content areas | Time focus | | | |
	Current situation	Therapy situation	Past developmental issues	Future planning issues
States and state cycles	Find triggers to entry into dreaded and problematic states, problems in having desired states, and triggers to starting and repeating maladaptive cycles.	Discuss how to achieve states of therapeutic work as contrasted to over- and undermodulated states.	Clarify the person whose state and state cycles may have been imitated, leading to unwanted identifications.	Plan how to prevent maladaptive cycle repetitions, learning to stabilize new, more adaptive states.
Conflicted topics and defensive controls	Clarify irrational beliefs and extreme emotional response to specific ideas as well as obstacles to clarity.	Explore how and why the patient stifles emotional and ideational expression of conflictual themes.	Examine reasons for irresolution on a theme and for forming habitual defensive styles and character traits.	Plan conscious counters to conditioned associations, automatic defensiveness, and unconscious avoidances.
Identity and relationships	Contrast rational views with erroneous self-judgments and irrational views of ways of affiliation with others.	Identify disagreements about patient-therapist roles. Contrast transference and countertransference with therapeutic roles, challenges, and integrations of discrepant attitudes.	Explore history of relationships and reasons for development of repertoire of self-schemas and role relationship models.	Encourage the patient as he or she tries out new affiliative and self-developmental procedures.

be inappropriate, these beliefs may have been reasonable or misunderstood in the past. Insight into their formations may be valuable in counteracting their continued operation.

Last is a focus on *future planning issues*. The aim of therapy is to improve the future; therefore, therapy progresses slowly toward this goal.

Foci of Attention in Therapy: External Orientation

☐ Symptoms and Problems

The social act of communicating our pain, distress, and fear of what will happen next is restorative if there is a resonance of empathic and benign understanding. Being well listened to can lead toward state stabilization. By naming the patient's unique individual experiences, we help. Our technique is to choose apt labels for experiences that our patient finds confusing, vague, and perhaps never-before-communicated. Sharing such labels increases the clarity and specificity of communications and increases our patient's sense of self-control.

We can explore how, when, and why these symptoms and problems limit life activities. Questions are asked and answered. Could a headache be a way of avoiding confrontation with others? Could procrastination occur when creative work is disappointing? We will perhaps find it valuable to avoid suggesting answers; we can instead convey our attitude as one of calm and gradual exploration in search of the truth.

Our ability to describe problems back to the patient can be considerably enhanced by observing analogous experiences to symptoms during therapy. These were called signs in the chapter on the first step of formulation, the selection and listing of phenomena. For example, an anxious patient may start to fidget restlessly, perhaps pulling at a lip and jiggling a leg during a therapy session. We can observe what topics evoke these limb movements. We may choose when and if to interpret the linkage between the meanings contemplated and the signs of increasing anxiety. We pay close attention to observing what memories and fantasies trigger more fidgeting. Then we can review past development and ask: How did this phenomenon of muscle tension and restless gesturing develop? When did it start? How has it changed with time?

We may then shift the time frame to the future. Both patient and therapist may describe what each expects will or could happen. What does the patient expect to happen if therapy works? What if it fails to work? The patient may expect total relief from all tension or distress. That expectation may be discrepant with our knowledge about what is realistically possible. We can clarify the situation.

☐ Recent Life Events

Symptoms may flare up or have a first onset after social or biological insults. Threats, separations, losses, and sharp changes in milieu, role, responsibility, or chemical intake may trigger a crisis. Increases in poverty, inequality, stigmatization, ethnic conflict, and physical ailments may make psychological coping with stress more difficult. Irrational explanations make defensive maneuvers more likely as rational coping begins to seem hopeless and the self is experienced as helpless.

Social changes may disrupt usually supportive friendships, affiliations, and loves. Separations and losses are common precipitants of increased symptoms. The effects of the death of a loved one, a divorce, or a violent assault may lead, eventually, to depression, inability to concentrate, and unbidden images. A promotion at work that adds high expectations and vexing responsibilities and reduces useful mentoring may occur before the onset of fatigue, anxiety, and sleeplessness. A patient may not fully recognize the connection. We can clarify small models of cause and effect.

One of our most important techniques is clarification and interpretation of the connections between external events and inner meanings that lead to personal meanings about the event. By clarifying the realistic and imagined implications of a recent event, we help a patient appraise crucial differences between reality and fantasy. For instance, a patient may attribute a sour mood to having just eaten the wrong foods rather than to unconsciously realizing this date is the anniversary of a loss. This differentiation of reality and fantasy is dangerous ground because it concerns psychological "reality," and the therapist does not know the exact truth. It is an area we must enter, however, alert to maintaining a "don't be too sure" attitude, and ready to check with others on "what is real," when that is essential to planning the treatment. For example, when the topic of attention concerns memories of a traumatic event, our patient may experience memories of what really happened as if the events depicted were unreal or may experience fantasy as if the events actually occurred. We may have to remain equidistant between the poles of actuality and imagination, not being sure, but knowing that all memory is constructed and constantly reconstructed (Schacter and Tulving 1994).

You may at times direct attention to the patient's expectations of stressful states in the treatment situation. How might the patient be expecting treatment to increase or reduce stress? To expose acts that are bad or embarrassing? To increase rather than decrease personal exposure and vulnerability?

A patient may want to express "repressed memories" and have you help reduce stress by hypnosis. This may run counter to the techniques you are actually likely to use. Other patients may expect therapy to increase stress, evoking memories that will lead to overwhelming emotional responses, exposing shameful action patterns the patient cannot stop, or sharpening longings that will remain frustrated. Less consciously, the same patient may expect you to repeat exploitative actions of other persons in previous real and fantasized traumas. A patient who has been abused may fear abuse from a therapist; one who has been scorned and abandoned may fear a repetition. By focusing conscious attention to such concerns, we gradually help a patient to confront fears consciously and voluntarily. We can help patients recognize what is going on and modify their irrational expectations. They may expect us to degrade and exploit them or to idealize and love them, but we remain ethical and expert, going to neither extreme of involvement.

We review the link between past and present to consider possible futures. We ask: How can the future be different? What steps can the patient take now in preparation to handle possible future crises? How can the patient plan to prevent acting out repetitions of past irrational beliefs in the future? Where in planning actions does the patient have residual doubt or confusion? Such questions lead to deeper contemplation of unresolved topics and to a gradual internal and personal focus on what can change.

☐ Current Dilemmas of Choice

About the current situation of pressure at work, a patient says: "I do not know whether to ask for a transfer, just do what I am told, or assert my objections to my boss. I get a headache just thinking about it." Even in the therapy situation, the patient has a dilemma: "Shall I talk about whether I want a transfer to another department, how to assert myself in this department, or whether my headaches could be a brain tumor?" We can help patients at this level by linking current external crises to internal beliefs and contradictions.

When stressful life events precipitate a mental disorder, we can focus first on getting a clear description of the patient's experience before, during, and after the symptoms appeared or trauma happened. Then we can focus on present and future concerns. What competing alternatives of choice does the patient face? Are there "damned if you do and damned if you don't" dilemmas? What beliefs support the pros and cons at any pole of choice? Why has it previously been difficult to arrive at rational choices? These questions deepen the process into concern for what can change internally, in the mind of the patient.

Foci of Attention in Therapy: Internal Orientation

☐ States and State Cycles

As therapy progresses, we usually observe that patients increase their ability to use thought and discourse, to contemplate before acting, and to act rather than becoming paralyzed with doubt. These changes increase abilities to tolerate emotion and uncertainty. Patients can then focus more deeply on obscured patterns. Once recognized, we notice these patterns again and again. Cycles of states can be clarified.

Knowing about the cycle leads to conscious anticipation of what might happen next. Such knowledge gives the patient a chance to brace the self. Triggers for dreaded and problematic states can be known in advance and confronted in ways that do not lead to the usual repetitions. Early preparation can interrupt hazardous later sequences in the cycle.

Once we clarify state cycles, it may be useful to find the reasons for repeating the pattern. As shown in Table 6–2, during therapy sessions, we can focus attention on identifying trigger events that cause shifts in state. We can show the patient differences between states in which useful information processing occurs and states that are either too resistant or undermodulated.

Then, turning to a past time frame, we can ask: Who else had states like this? Whom may you have imitated? Turning to a future time frame, we help the patient prevent repetition of self-impairing state cycles and practice ways to stabilize new, more adaptive states.

Here is an illustration of state analysis. Mr. Brown was married, and he worked at a rewarding and demanding position. He came to see me because of anxious and depressive symptoms that did not clearly meet any DSM-IV (American Psychiatric Association 1994) Axis I diagnosis. These were real symptoms, but he used them as a kind of ticket of admission to psychotherapy. After initial sessions, he revealed a perverse behavior. He was worried that his wife might divorce him if he did not get help to prevent actions that she saw as strange and disgusting behavior. He masturbated using her underwear as a kind of fetish object. She had recently, for the first time, caught him in the act.

He would rub himself with her garment and achieve orgasm, but then feel guilty. When his wife found him, he felt mortified. In a confusing way, he also became very angry with her. When she brought up the incident repeatedly, he shifted into an undermodulated rage, which then led to more shame and guilt because it seemed so unjustified.

Mr. Brown had been too ashamed to describe this problem during early interviews. But after a few sessions of psychotherapy focused on why he was anxious and depressed, he progressed to states in which his shame was tolerable in a shimmering state of mind. Our level of focus moved to an internal orientation, as in Table 6–2. After his revelation, we were able to examine an illuminating cycle of his states.

His act of masturbating with his wife's underwear was related to his early erotic experiences, which involved both pleasurable bodily arousal and fear. He had a symbolic or screen memory of suddenly opening the door to his mother's room when she was undressing. She whipped him in the face with a piece of her underwear. A metal fitting cut his eye. Being whipped by his angry mother was frightening, but the experience had an erotic component. Women's underwear became an erotic fetish in his adult life. He could not control a woman, but he could control the garment. The trauma to his face was not going to occur again, but the sense of danger was thrilling.

We focused our attention in therapy on his tense and anxious state of mind, in the current time frame. He felt compelled to relieve this state by masturbating with his wife's underwear. It seemed so odd because they had a mutually satisfying sex life. By masturbating with her underwear, he was able to shift from an anxious state to a thrilled state. This thrilled state contrasted with an anxiously erotic state that he had during sexual mutuality with his wife. Although aroused with her, he felt tense about her possible eruptive actions. He described becoming frightened during a recent episode of intercourse with his wife when she expressed the passion of an orgasm. It seemed to him that she was selfishly preoccupied with her own pleasure, losing concern for him. She could become a large woman thrashing around in bed, possibly hurting him. This idea seemed preposterous to him, but it seemed linked directly to his fear.

Mr. Brown also had depressive states in which he felt sour, apathetic, and empty. In the current situation, these states were triggered whenever his wife left him for an evening each week for social activities with her friends. He recalled such sour states in the past, when his mother was either depressed or preoccupied. He experienced a similar state when I had to answer the phone, cancel an appointment, or leave on vacation.

Before he married, Mr. Brown counteracted a sour state by engaging in the thrilling activity of masturbation. The use of women's underwear helped him get aroused and aided his mental imagery of a sexy woman. The underwear and the imagery were controlled by his own will, "not her selfishness." The underwear was safer than a woman. After marriage, he also used this activity, and his wife's underwear, when he felt tense. I encouraged him to notice when he first felt tension and to tolerate or deal with it without his familiar but clandestine activity, to prevent the end-point states of guilt or undermodulated rage.

The masturbatory, fetishistic activity was a special state of mind. It helped Mr. Brown achieve erotic satisfaction, but it was even more important as a way to relieve a dreaded state of feeling *empty, sour, and depressed* or an *anxious state of fear of loss of contact* with a person he believed he needed to have present at all times. The erotic masturbatory state, achieved alone, was a quasi-adaptive compromise to avoid the dangers of a wish-fear dilemma between a desired erotic state in interaction with a partner, and the fear the partner would take over or leave him. Some of his states and beliefs are summarized in Figure 6–1 and Figure 6–2.

Problematic compromise	Quasi-adaptive compromise
• Anxious, fearful	• Erotic masturbatory
• Empty, depressed	• Erotic interactive
Dreaded	**Desired**

Figure 6–1.   Configuration of states for Mr. Brown.

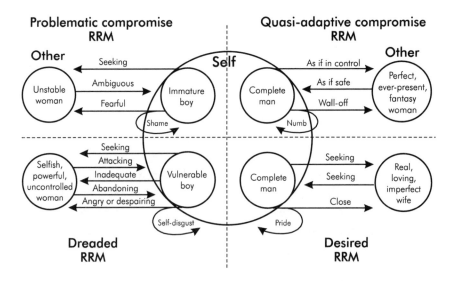

Figure 6–2.   Role relationship model (RRM) configuration for Mr. Brown.

Mr. Brown was then able to confront the sense of identity and patterns of interpersonal relationships in each of these states. Eventually, he felt a reduction in anxiety and depression. He gained a sense of safe closeness with his wife, even during passionate erotic activities. He gave up his fetishistic acts. He could tolerate being alone without shifting into a sense of empty identity.

☐ Conflicted Topics and Defensive Controls

Signs of defensive control processes and signs of emerging but stifled emotions may signal which themes are important, conflicted, and unresolved. Conflicted topics may include unintegrated memories and fantasies, dissociated views of identity, thwarted ambitions, incomplete tasks, wish-driven fantasies, and discrepant attitudes about what to do next. The habitual defensive controls that act as obstacles to clarity on these themes, and so as obstacles to therapy, may be counteracted by suggesting how to focus attention, thought, and discourse or by interpreting of resistances in treatment. Through conscious efforts, a patient may gradually be able to modify habitual avoidances and distortions. Life choices that have been avoided may now be made.

We often see regressive states during therapy. These states contain raw emotions and impulses. They may include self-loathing to the point of revulsion, compensatory grandiosity, revenge, and magical thinking. We usually try to restore equilibrium and prevent such regressions. Sometimes, however, we encourage them for exploratory purposes. Work at this level means reducing defenses. The raw emotions that may then be expressed go beyond the mind of the patient and affect the emotional reactivity of the therapist. Complex intersubjective states may occur. These require of us a careful self-analysis to reduce the effects of countertransference. Only some patients can integrate experiences from their regressive states, and encouraging these states can be dangerous to many patients. Advanced training is required before the therapist can feel truly confident in knowing how and when to promote regressive experiences.

☐ Identity and Relationships

As the patient becomes attentive to states, it is possible to clarify the views of self and other that tend to occur in each state. Then we can interpret shifts in identity and role relationship models to explain when, how, and why shifts in state occur. A patient, by focusing attention on views of self and others, can come to see what is usually obscure: internal, enduring contradictions, conflicts, and discrepancies in beliefs. This insight leads toward an integration of contradictions and to the gradual development of the umbrella-like, supraordinate schemas discussed in the preceding chapter. We help patients establish associational linkages between alternative views to help them form such integrations in self-organization.

New schemas may gain priority over previous immature, maladaptive, and regressive ones. At first, new intentions may have to be conscious and deliberate. Then, with time, new schemas and integrations become automatic. Our patient gains poise. State transitions become smooth rather than explosive. We can help by clarifying and interpreting the major discrepancies between ideal, actual, dreaded, and desired views of self. We help patients examine past and present sources of identity and a concern for "future selves," imagining what can happen.

Discords between what is expected of others and what they actually do are also useful foci of attention. We may find it useful to explore critic roles, in which the observing self evaluates the activities and intentions of the self as agent of action. Harsh, self-critical, self-monitoring can be compared with more accepting values. The result can reduce the frequency and intensity of states of shame, guilt, and self-disgust.

By examining together the history of past relationships, we can help our patient develop an internal story that grows in consistency and acceptance. A sense of continuity helps many patients integrate various self-concepts into a sense of identity that feels stable and coherent rather than fragile and fragmentary. As we question how enduring attitudes formed and recurred in the past, we encourage a reexamination of these attitudes in the present. We help our patient consider chances for new behaviors in the future. We can ask: Did the patient adopt or rebel against the affirming or prohibiting attitudes presented by another person? Did he or she like or dislike a parent, sibling, or significant other?

Hitherto forgotten memories and fantasies from childhood may emerge. More often, long-recalled episodes seem to fit together more and more. Even bad memories are better tolerated in a container of discourse that involves two communicating adult minds rather than one mind of a possibly overwhelmed and confused child.

Review of traumatic memories and fantasies may help clarify a script of wishes linked to feared consequences. The patient may then plan trials of new relationship patterns based on these motives. By carrying out new patterns that are repeatedly successfully, he or she can forge new schematizations. As these new schemas become the dominant organized knowledge structures, behavior will become more automatic, and it will require less volitional effort. Until then, heightened levels of awareness of self and self-control are indicated.

The therapist and patient analyze each new crisis and difficult situation to find contradictions in views of self and others, negative emotions, and conflicted intentions. They clarify discrepant views of self and others. Both seek to speak of new, better concepts.

Therapy may provide the patient with a new relationship experience. We may define our characteristics with our patient, and both parties' transactional patterns within a therapeutic alliance. One possible version of the safe, ethical, and effective features in such a possibly novel relationship for the patient is shown in Figure 6–3. Stating the realistic basis of these features can form a schema for patients deficient in experiences of trust.

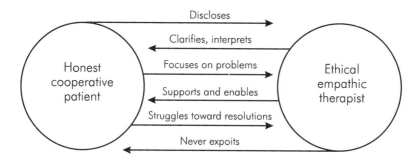

Figure 6–3. Role relationship model of a therapeutic alliance may become a new schema.

Summary

The first four steps of case formulation involve the selection and explanation of phenomena, the clarification of states and cycles, the identification of topics of concern and defensive control processes, and inferences about conflictual or reality-discrepant identity and relationship schemas. The fifth and final step integrates these foci and explanations with treatment plans. This process often leads to a technique that starts with complaints and moves toward ways to modify dysfunctional beliefs, irrational processes, and conflictual attitudes. That modification is up to the patient. By offering a readiness to look to the future and the past as well as examine the present, we help our patients voyage through time in a safe space.

REFERENCES

Allen JG: Ego states and object relations. Bull Menninger Clin 41:522–538, 1977

Allport F: Theories of Perception and the Concept of Structure. New York, John Wiley, 1955

American Psychiatric Association: Diagnostic and Statistical Manual of Mental Disorders, 3rd Edition. Washington, DC, American Psychiatric Association, 1980

American Psychiatric Association: Diagnostic and Statistical Manual of Mental Disorders, 4th Edition. Washington, DC, American Psychiatric Association, 1994

Arlow J: Unconscious fantasy and disturbances of conscious experiences. Psychoanal Q 38:1–27, 1969

Ashby WR: Design for a Brain, 1st Edition. New York, John Wiley, 1952

Ashby WR: Design for a Brain: The Origin of Adaptive Behavior, 2nd Edition. New York, John Wiley, 1960

Bartlett FC: Remembering: A Study in Experimental and Social Psychology. Cambridge, England, Cambridge University Press, 1932

Basch MF: Psychoanalysis and theory formation. Annual of Psychoanalysis 1:39–52, 1973

Beck AT: Cognitive Therapy and Emotional Disorders. New York, International Universities Press, 1976

Beck AT: Cognitive models of depression. Journal of Cognitive Psychotherapy: An International Quarterly 1:5–37, 1987

Beck JS: Cognitive Therapy: Basics and Beyond. New York, Guilford, 1995

Beitman BD, Goldfried MR, Norcross JC: The movement toward integrating the psychotherapies: an overview. Am J Psychiatry 146:138–147, 1989

Benjamin LS, Friedrich FJ: Contributions of Structural Analysis of Social Behavior (SASB) to the bridge between cognitive science and a science of object relations, in Person Schemas and Maladaptive Interpersonal Patterns. Edited by Horowitz MJ. Chicago, IL, University of Chicago Press, 1991, pp 379–412

Berne E: Transactional Analysis in Psychotherapy. New York, Grove Press, 1961

Berne E: Games People Play. New York, Grove Press, 1964

Berne E: What Do You Say After You Say Hello? The Psychology of Human Destiny. New York, Grove Press, 1972

Bowlby J: Attachment and Loss, Vol 1: Attachment. New York, Basic Books, 1969

Bowlby J: Developmental psychology comes of age. Am J Psychiatry 145:1–10, 1988

Carr V: The concept of clinical state in psychiatry: a review. Compr Psychiatry 24:370–391, 1983

Caston J: Can analysts agree? the problems of consensus and the psychoanalytic mannequin. J Am Psychoanal Assoc 41:493–548, 1993

Conte H, Plutchik R (eds): Ego Defenses: Theory and Measurement. New York, John Wiley, 1994

Cook TD: A quasi-sampling theory of the generalization of casual relationships, in Understanding Causes and Generalizing About Them. Edited by Sechrest L, Scott AG. San Francisco, CA, Jossey-Bass, 1993

Dixon NF: Preconscious Processing. New York, John Wiley, 1981

Docherty J, VanKammen DP, Siris SG, et al: Stages of onset of schizophrenic psychosis. Am J Psychiatry 135:420–426, 1978

Eells TD, Horowitz MJ, Singer J, et al: The role relationship models method: a comparison of independently derived case formulations. Psychotherapy Research 5:161–175, 1995

Ekman P, Davidson RJ (eds): The Nature of Emotion. New York, Oxford University Press, 1994

Engle GL: The clinical application of the biopsychosocial model. Am J Psychiatry 137:535–544, 1980

Erikson E: The dream specimen of psychoanalysis. J Am Psychoanal Assoc 4:56–121, 1954

Fairbairn WR: An Object Relations Theory of the Personality. New York, Basic Books, 1954

Federn P: Ego Psychology and the Psychoses. New York, Basic Books, 1952

Freud A: The Ego and Mechanisms of Defense. New York, International Universities Press, 1936

Freud S: The interpretation of dreams (1900), in The Standard Edition of the Complete Psychological Works of Sigmund Freud, Vol 3. Translated and edited by Strachey J. London, Hogarth Press, 1955

Freud S: On psychoanalysis (1903), in The Standard Edition of the Complete Psychological Works of Sigmund Freud, Vol 12. Translated and edited by Strachey J. London, Hogarth Press, 1964, pp 205–211

Freud S: Three essays on the theory of sexuality (1905), in The Standard Edition of the Complete Psychological Works of Sigmund Freud. Translated and edited by Strachey J. London, Hogarth Press, 1953, pp 125–144

Freud S: The dynamics of the transference (1912a), in The Standard Edition of the Complete Psychological Works of Sigmund Freud, Vol 12. Translated and edited by Strachey J. London, Hogarth Press, 1958, pp 97–108

Freud S: Recommendations to physicians practicing psycho-analysis (1912b), in The Standard Edition of the Complete Psychological Works of Sigmund Freud, Vol 12. Translated and edited by Strachey J. London, Hogarth Press, 1958, pp 109–120

Freud S: On beginning the treatment: further recommendations on the technique of psycho-analysis I (1913), in The Standard Edition of the Complete Psychological Works of Sigmund Freud, Vol 12. Translated and edited by Strachey J. London, Hogarth Press, 1958, pp 121–144

Freud S: Remembering, repeating, and working-through: further recommendations on the technique of psycho-analysis II (1914), in The Standard Edition of the Complete Psychological Works of Sigmund Freud, Vol 12. Translated and edited by Strachey J. London, Hogarth Press, 1958, pp 145–156

Freud S: The ego and id (1923), in The Standard Edition of the Complete Psychological Works of Sigmund Freud, Vol 19. Translated and edited by Strachey J. London, Hogarth Press, 1961, pp 1–66

Freud S: Inhibition, symptoms and anxiety (1926), in The Standard Edition of the Complete Psychological Works of Sigmund Freud, Vol 19. Translated and edited by Strachey J. London, Hogarth Press, 1955, pp 87–156

Gaarter K: Control of states of consciousness, attainment through external feedback augmenting control of psychophysiological variables. Arch Gen Psychiatry 25:436–441, 1971

Gedo J, Goldberg A: Models of the Mind. Chicago, IL, University of Chicago Press, 1973

Goldfried MR: Toward a common language for case formulation. Journal of Psychotherapy Integration 5:221–244, 1996

Goldsmith SR, Mandel AJ: The dynamic formulation: a critique of a psychiatric ritual. Am J Psychiatry 125:1738–1743, 1969

Greenacre P: Trauma, Growth and Personality. New York, WW Norton, 1952

Horowitz MJ: Art therapy, in Handbook of Psychiatric Therapies. Edited by Masserman J. Chicago, IL, Science House, 1973, pp 156–162

Horowitz MJ: Diagnosis and treatment of stress response syndromes: general principles, in Emergency Mental Health and Disaster Aid Services. Edited by Parad H. New York, Prentice-Hall, 1976

Horowitz MJ: Image Formation and Cognition. New York, Appleton-Century-Crofts, 1978

Horowitz MJ: States of Mind: Configurational Analysis of Individual Psychology. New York, Plenum, 1979/1987

Horowitz MJ: Levels of interpretation in dynamic psychotherapy. Psychoanalytic Psychology 3:39–45, 1986

Horowitz MJ: Introduction to Psychodynamics: A New Synthesis. New York, Basic Books, 1988a

Horowitz MJ (ed): Psychodynamics and Cognition. Chicago, IL, University of Chicago Press, 1988b

Horowitz MJ: Relationship schema formulation: role-relationship models and intrapsychic conflict. Psychiatry 52:260–274, 1989

Horowitz MJ (ed): Person Schemas and Maladaptive Interpersonal Patterns. Chicago, IL, University of Chicago Press, 1991a

Horowitz MJ: Psychic structure and the processes of change, in Hysterical Personality Style and the Histrionic Personality Disorder, 2nd Edition. Edited by Horowitz MJ. Northvale, NJ, Jason Aronson, 1991b, pp 193–261

Horowitz MJ: Defensive control of states and person schemas. J Am Psychoanal Assoc 41:67–89, 1993

Horowitz MJ: Configurational analysis and the use of role relationship models to understand transference. Psychotherapy Research 3:184–196, 1994

Horowitz MJ: Histrionic personality disorder, in Treatment of Psychiatric Disorders, 2nd Edition. Edited by Gabbard G. Washington, DC, American Psychiatric Press, 1995a, pp 2311–2326

Horowitz MJ: Organizational levels of self and other schematizations, in Personality Development. Edited by Westenberg P, Rogers A, Cohn L, et al. Hillsdale, NJ, Lawrence Erlbaum Associates, 1995b

Horowitz MJ: Stress Response Syndromes, 3rd Edition. Northvale, NJ, Jason Aronson, 1997

Horowitz MJ: Cognitive psychodynamics: the clinical use of states, persons schemas, and defensive control process theory, in Cognitive Science and the Unconscious. Edited by Stein D. Washington, DC, American Psychiatric Press (in press)

Horowitz MJ, Becker SS: Cognitive response to stress: experimental studies of "a compulsion to repeat trauma," in Psychoanalysis and Contemporary Science, Vol 1. Edited by Holt R, Peterfreund E. New York, Macmillan, 1972, pp 258–305

Horowitz MJ, Eells T: Case formulation using role-relationship model configurations: a reliability study. Psychotherapy Research 3:57–68, 1993

Horowitz MJ, Stinson CH: Defenses as aspects of person schemas and control processes, in Ego Defenses: Theory and Measurement. Edited by Conte H, Plutchik R. New York, John Wiley, 1994, pp 79–97

Horowitz MJ, Stinson CH: Consciousness and processes of control. Journal of Psychotherapy Practice and Research 4:123–139, 1995

Horowitz MJ, Marmar C, Krupnick J, et al: Personality Styles and Brief Psychotherapy. New York, Basic Books, 1984a

Horowitz MJ, Marmar C, Weiss D, et al: Brief psychotherapy of bereavement reactions: the relationship of process to outcome. Arch Gen Psychiatry 41:438–448, 1984b

Horowitz MJ, Markman HC, Stinson CH, et al: A classification theory of defense, in Repression and Dissociation: Implications for Personality Theory, Psychopathology, and Health. Edited by Singer J. Chicago, IL, University of Chicago Press, 1990, pp 61–84

Horowitz MJ, Cooper S, Fridhandler B, et al: Control processes and defense mechanisms. Journal of Psychotherapy Practice and Research 1:324–336, 1992

Horowitz MJ, Milbrath C, Reidbord S, et al: Elaboration and dyselaboration: measures of expression and defense in discourse. Psychotherapy Research 3:278–293, 1993a

Horowitz MJ, Stinson CH, Fridhandler B, et al: Pathological grief: an intensive case study. Psychiatry 56:356–374, 1993b

Horowitz MJ, Stinson C, Curtis D, et al: Topics and signs: defensive control of emotional expression. J Consult Clin Psychol 61:421–430, 1993c

Horowitz MJ, Milbrath C, Ewert M, et al: Cyclical patterns of states of mind in psychotherapy. Am J Psychiatry 151:1767–1770, 1994a

Horowitz MJ, Milbrath C, Jordan D, et al: Expressive and defensive behavior during discourse of unresolved topics: a single case study. J Pers 62:527–563, 1994b

Horowitz MJ, Znoj H, Stinson CH: Defensive control processes: use of theory in research, formulation, and therapy of stress response syndromes, in Handbook of Coping. Edited by Zeidner M, Endler N. New York, John Wiley, 1995a, pp 532–553

Horowitz MJ, Eells T, Singer J, et al: Role relationship models for case formulation. Arch Gen Psychiatry 53:627–632, 1995b

Horowitz MJ, Milbrath C, Stinson C: Signs of defensive control locate conflicted topics in discourse. Arch Gen Psychiatry 52:1040–1057, 1995c

Horowitz MJ, Stinson CH, Milbrath C: Role relationship models: a person schematic method for inferring beliefs about identity and social action, in Essays on Ethnography and Human Development. Edited by Colby A, Jessor R, Schweder R. Chicago, IL, University of Chicago Press, 1996, pp 253–274

Horowitz MJ, Eells T, Singer J, et al: Role relationship models for case formulation of personality disorders, in Cognition and Psychodynamics. Edited by Kurtzman H. New York, Oxford University Press (in press)

Janet P: The Major Symptoms of Hysteria. New York, Hafner, 1965

Jaspers J: The phenomenological approach in psychopathology. Br J Psychiatry 114:1313–1323, 1968

Jung CG: The Integration of Personality. New York, Farrar & Rinehart, 1939

Kelly GA: The Psychology of Personal Constructs, Vols 1 & 2. New York, WW Norton, 1955

Kernberg O: The treatment of patients with borderline personality disorders. Int J Psychoanal 49:600–619, 1968

Kernberg O: Borderline Conditions and Pathological Narcissism. Northvale, NJ, Jason Aronson, 1975

Kernberg O: Object Relations Theory and Clinical Psychoanalysis. Northvale, NJ,, Jason Aronson, 1976

Klein M: Contributions to Psychoanalysis. London, Hogarth Press, 1948

Kohut H: Restoration of the Self. New York, International Universities Press, 1977

Kosslyn SM, Koenig O: Wet Mind: The New Cognitive Neuroscience. New York, Free Press, 1992

Kovacs M, Beck A: Maladaptive cognitive structures in depression. Am J Psychiatry 135:325–333, 1978

Kuhl J, Beckmann J: Historical perspectives in the study of action control, in Action Control: From Cognition to Behavior. Edited by Kuhl J, Beckmann J. New York, Springer-Verlag, 1985, pp 89–121

Kurtzman H (ed): Cognition and Psychodynamics: New Perspectives. New York, Oxford University Press (in press)

Lazare A: Hidden conceptual models in clinical psychiatry. N Engl J Med 299:345–351, 1973

Lazare A: A multidimensional approach to psychopathology in outpatient psychiatry, in Diagnosis and Treatment, 2nd Edition. Edited by Lazare A. Baltimore, MD, Williams & Wilkins, 1989, pp 7–16

Lazarus RS: Emotion and Adaptation. New York, Oxford University Press, 1991

Lewin K: A Dynamic Theory of Personality. New York, McGraw-Hill, 1935

Lichtenberg JD: The development of the sense of self. J Am Psychoanal Assoc 23:453–484, 1975

Luborsky L: Principles of Psychoanalytic Psychotherapy: A Manual for Supportive Expressive Treatment. New York, Basic Books, 1984

Luborsky L, Crits-Christoph P (eds): Understanding Transference: The CCRT Method. New York, Basic Books, 1990

Markus H: Self-schemata and processing information about the self. J Pers Soc Psychol 35:63–78, 1977

McWilliams N: Psychoanalytic Diagnosis: Understanding Personality Structure in the Clinical Process. New York, Guilford, 1994

Miller GA, Galanter E, Pribram KH: Plans and the Structure of Behavior. New York, Holt, 1960

Murray HA: Explorations in Personality. New York, Oxford University Press, 1938

Palmer SE: PDP: a new paradigm for cognitive theory. Contemporary Psychology 32:925–928, 1987

Perry C, Augusto F, Cooper S: Assessing psychodynamic conflicts: reliability of the ideographic conflict formulation method. Psychiatry 52:289–301, 1989

Perry J: Use of longitudinal data to validate personality disorders, in Personality Disorders: New Perspectives on Diagnostic Validity (Progress in Psychiatry No. 20). Edited by Oldham JM. Washington, DC, American Psychiatric Press, 1991, pp 24–40

Perry JC, Cooper SH: An empirical study of defense mechanisms: clinical interview and life vignette ratings. Arch Gen Psychiatry 46:444–452, 1989

Perry S, Cooper AM, Michels R: The psychodynamic formulation: its purpose, structure, and clinical application. Am J Psychiatry 144:543–550, 1987

Persons JB: A case formulations approach to cognitive-behavior therapy: application to panic disorder. Psychiatric Annals 22:470–473, 1992

Persons JB: Case conceptualizations in cognitive-behavior therapy, in Cognitive Therapies in Action: Evolving Innovative Practice. Edited by Kuehlwein KT, Rosen H. San Francisco, CA, Jossey-Bass, 1993, pp 33–53

Piaget J: The Child's Conception of Physical Causality. New York, Harcourt Brace, 1930

Piper WE, Azim HF, Joyce AS, et al: Transference interpretations, therapeutic alliance, and outcome in short-term individual psychotherapy. Arch Gen Psychiatry 48:946–953, 1991

Posner MI (ed): Foundations of Cognitive Science. Cambridge, MA, MIT Press, 1989

Reich W: Character Analysis. New York, Noonday Press, 1949

Rumelhart DE, McClelland JL (eds): Parallel Distributed Processing: Exploration in the Microstructures of Cognition, Vols 1 & 2. Cambridge, MA, MIT Press, 1986

Sandler J: The background of safety. Int J Psychoanal 41:352–356, 1960

Schacter D, Tulving E (eds): Memory Systems. Cambridge, MA, MIT Press, 1994

Shapiro D: Neurotic Styles. New York, Basic Books, 1965

Silberschatz G, Curtis J, Sampson H, et al: Mt. Zion Hospital and Medical Center: research on the process of change in psychotherapy, in Psychotherapy Research: An International Review of Programmatic Studies. Edited by Beutler L, Crago M. Washington, DC, American Psychological Association Press, 1991, pp 56–64

Singer JL: Beyond repression and the defenses, in Repression and Dissociation: Implications for Personality Theory, Psychopathology, and Health. Edited by Singer J. Chicago, IL, University of Chicago Press, 1990

Singer JL, Salovey P: Organized knowledge structures and personality, in Person Schemas and Maladaptive Interpersonal Patterns. Edited by Horowitz MJ. Chicago, IL, University of Chicago Press, 1991, pp 33–80

Slap JW, Saykin AJ: The schema: basic concept in a nonmetapsychological model of the mind. Psychoanalysis and Contemporary Thought 6:305–325, 1983

Sperry L, Gudeman J, Blackwell B, et al: Psychiatric Case Formulations. Washington, DC, American Psychiatric Press, 1992

Squire LR: Mechanisms of memory. Science 232:1612–1619, 1986

Stein D (ed): Cognitive Science and the Unconscious. Washington, DC, American Psychiatric Press (in press)

Stinson CH, Horowitz MJ: Psyclops: an exploratory graphical system for clinical research and education. Psychiatry 56:375–389, 1993

Stinson CH, Palmer S: Parallel distributed processing models of person schemas and psychopathologies, in Person Schemas and Maladaptive Interpersonal Patterns. Edited by Horowitz MJ. Chicago, IL, University of Chicago Press, 1991, pp 339–378

Strupp HH, Binder JL: Psychotherapy in a New Key. New York, Basic Books, 1984

Tomkins S: Script theory: differential magnification of affects, in Nebraska Symposium on Motivation, Vol 26. Edited by Howe H. Lincoln, University of Nebraska Press, 1978, pp 201–236

Turkat ID, Wolpe L: A behavioral formulation of clinical cases, in Behavioral Case Formulations. Edited by Turkat ID. New York, Harper & Row, 1988

Uleman JS, Bargh JA (eds): Unintended Thought. New York, Guilford, 1989

Vaillant G: Ego Mechanisms of Defense in Clinical and in Empirical Research. Washington, DC, American Psychiatric Press, 1992

Vaillant G: The Wisdom of Ego. Cambridge, MA, Harvard University Press, 1993

Wallerstein R: Forty-Two Lives in Treatment. New York, Guilford, 1986

Weed LL: Medical Records, Medical Education, and Patient Care: The Problem-Oriented Record as a Basic Tool. Cleveland, OH, Press of Case Western Reserve University, 1969

Wegner D, Pennebaker J (eds): Handbook of Mental Control. New York, Prentice-Hall, 1992

Weiss J: Bernfeld's "The facts of observation in psychoanalysis": a response from psychoanalytic research. Psychoanal Q 64:699–716, 1995

Weiss J, Sampson H (eds): The Psychoanalytic Process: Theory, Clinical Observation and Empirical Research. New York, Guilford, 1986

Winnicott DW: Transitional objects and transitional phenomena. Int J Psychoanal 43:89–97, 1953

World Health Organization: The ICD-10 Classification of Mental and Behavioural Disorders: Clinical Descriptions and Diagnostic Guidelines. Geneva, Switzerland, World Health Organization, 1992

Young JE: Cognitive Therapy for Personality Disorders: A Schema-Focussed Approach. Sarasota, FL, Professional Research Exchange, 1990

Zeidner M, Endler NH: Handbook of Coping. New York, John Wiley, 1995

INDEX